Amazing Keto Vegetarian Recipes

Simple and Delicious Plant-Based Ketogenic Diet Recipes to Lose Weight Easily and Feel Great

Lidia Wong

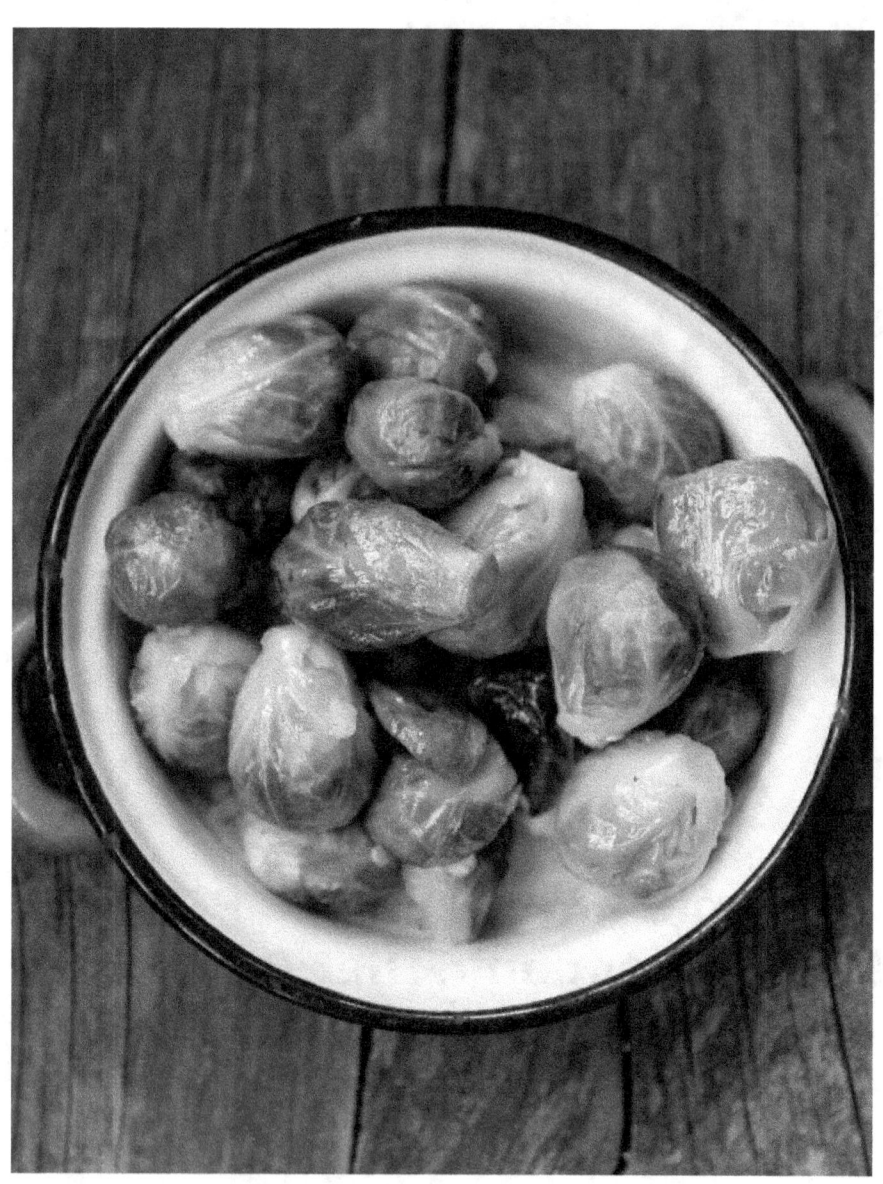

© **Copyright 2021 by Lidia Wong - All rights reserved.**

The content contained within this book may not be reproduced, duplicated or transmitted without direct written permission from the author or the publisher.
Under no circumstances will any blame or legal responsibility be held against the publisher, or author, for any damages, reparation, or monetary loss due to the information contained within this book. Either directly or indirectly.

Legal Notice:
This book is copyright protected. This book is only for personal use. You cannot amend, distribute, sell, use, quote or paraphrase any part, or the content within this book, without the consent of the author or publisher.

Disclaimer Notice:
Please note the information contained within this document is for educational and entertainment purposes only. All effort has been executed to present accurate, up to date, and reliable, complete information. No warranties of any kind are declared or implied. Readers acknowledge that the author is not engaging in the rendering of legal, financial, medical or professional advice. The content within this book has been derived from various sources. Please consult a licensed professional before attempting any techniques outlined in this book.
By reading this document, the reader agrees that under no circumstances is the author responsible for any losses, direct or indirect, which are incurred as a result of the use of information contained within this document, including, but not limited to, — errors, omissions, or inaccuracies.

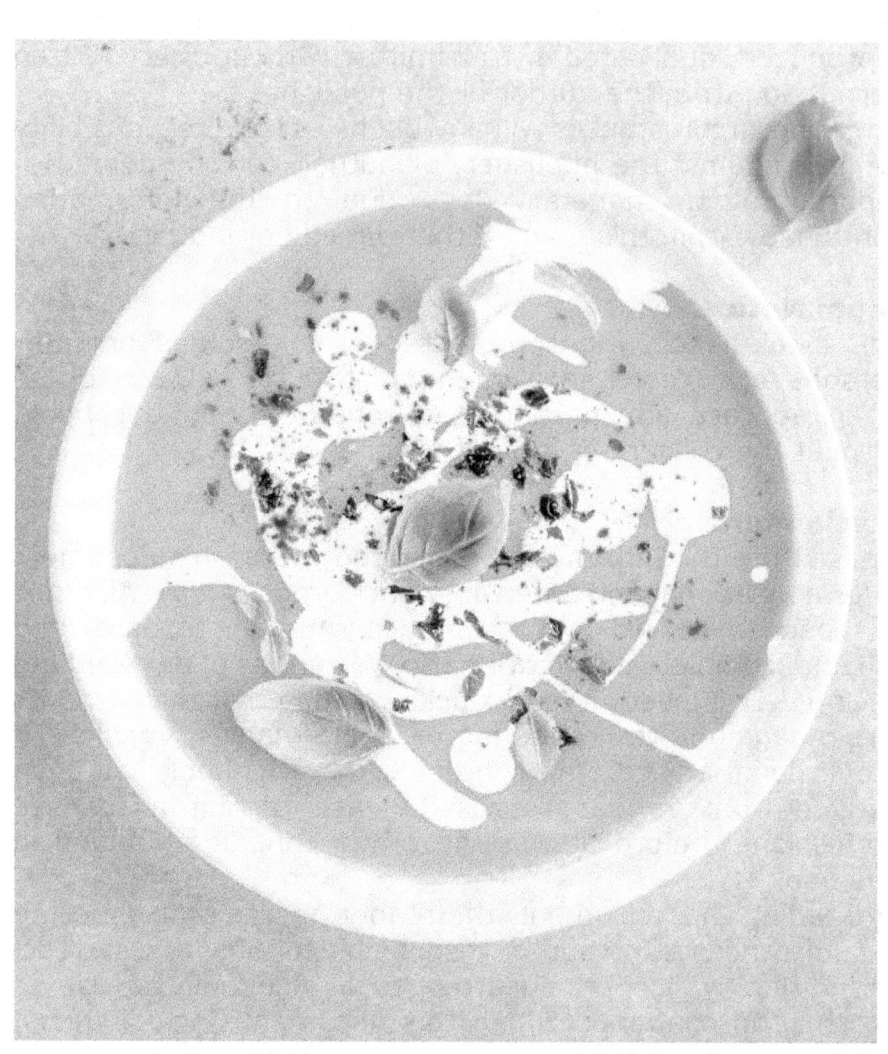

TABLE OF CONTENTS

INTRODUCTION 1

Coconut Waffles 3

Vanilla Chia Breakfast Pudding 5

Classic French Toasts 7

Avocado and Kale Soup 10

Minty Arugula Soup 11

Grapes, Avocado and Spinach Salad 12

Vinegar Cucumber, Olives and Shallots Salad 14

Parsley Chard Salad 15

Avocado, Endive and Asparagus Mix 17

Keto Taco Skillet 18

Vietnamese "Vermicelli" Salad 20

Simple Garlic Cauliflower Couscous 22

Mushroom Curry Pie 23

Green Avocado Carbonara 26

Herbed Zucchinis and Olives 29

Veggie Pan 31

Beet and Cabbage 33

Broccoli with Brussels Sprouts 35

Tomato Salad 37

Cinnamon-Scented Quinoa 39

Spinach and Kale Mix 41

Celery Soup 42

Spinach Soup 44

Alfalfa Sprouts Salad 46

Fried Okra 48

Avocado Broccoli Soup 50

Carrot Soup 52

Zucchini Soup 54

Almond Soup With Cardamom 56

Squash Soup With Pecans And Ginger 58

Balsamic Lentil Stew 60

Pumpkin-Pear Soup 62

Spicy Pinto Bean Soup 64

Puttanesca Seitan And Spinach Salad 66

Carrot And Orange Salad With Cashews And Cilantro 68

Dazzling Vegetable Salad 70

Indonesian Green BeanSalad With Cabbage And Carrots 72

Red Cabbage Slaw With Black-Vinegar Dressing 74

Cranberry-Carrot Salad 76

Mediterranean Quinoa Salad 77

Marinated Mushroom Wraps... 79

Macadamia-Cashew Patties...81

Peppermint-Cilantro Artichoke Hearts 83

Carrot Cake Bites... 85

Minty Fruit Salad.. 87

Avocado and Strawberries Salad 89

Mint Avocado Bars 90

Coconut milk smoothie 91

Keto Lemon Fat Bombs... 93

Chia Squares... 95

Mint Rice Pudding 97

Mug Cake... 99

NOTE **101**

INTRODUCTION

The keto diet is the shortened term for ketogenic diet and it is essentially a high-fat and low-carb diet that helps you lose weight, thereby bringing various health benefits. This diet drastically restricts your carb intake while increasing your fat intake; this pushes your body to go into a state know as "*ketosis*". We will tackle ketosis in a bit.

The human body uses glucose from carbs to fuel metabolic pathways—meaning various bodily functions like digestion, breathing, etc.. Essentially, anything that needs energy. Even when you are resting, the body needs fuel or energy for you to continue living. If you think about it, when have you ever stopped breathing, or your heart stopped beating, or your liver stopped from cleansing the body, or your kidneys from filtering blood?

Never, unless you're dead, which is the only time in which the body doesn't need energy. In normal circumstances, glucose is the primary pathway when it comes to sourcing the body's energy.

But the body also has another pathway; it can utilize fats to fuel the various bodily processes. And this is what we call "*ketosis*". And the body can only enter ketosis when there is no glucose available, thus the reason for sticking to a low-carb diet is essential in the keto diet. Since no glucose is available, the body is pushed to use fats—it can either come from the food you consume or from your body's fat reserves—the adipose tissue or from the flabby parts of your body. This is how the keto diet helps you lose weight, by burning up all those stored fats that you have and using it to fuel bodily processes.

That said, if for whatever reason you are a vegetarian, following a ketogenic diet can be extremely difficult. A vegetarian diet is largely free of animal products, which means that food tends to be usually high in carbohydrates. Still, with careful planning, it is possible. This Cookbook will provide you with various easy and delicious dishes to help you stick to your ketogenic diet plan while being a vegetarian.

Enjoy!

Coconut Waffles

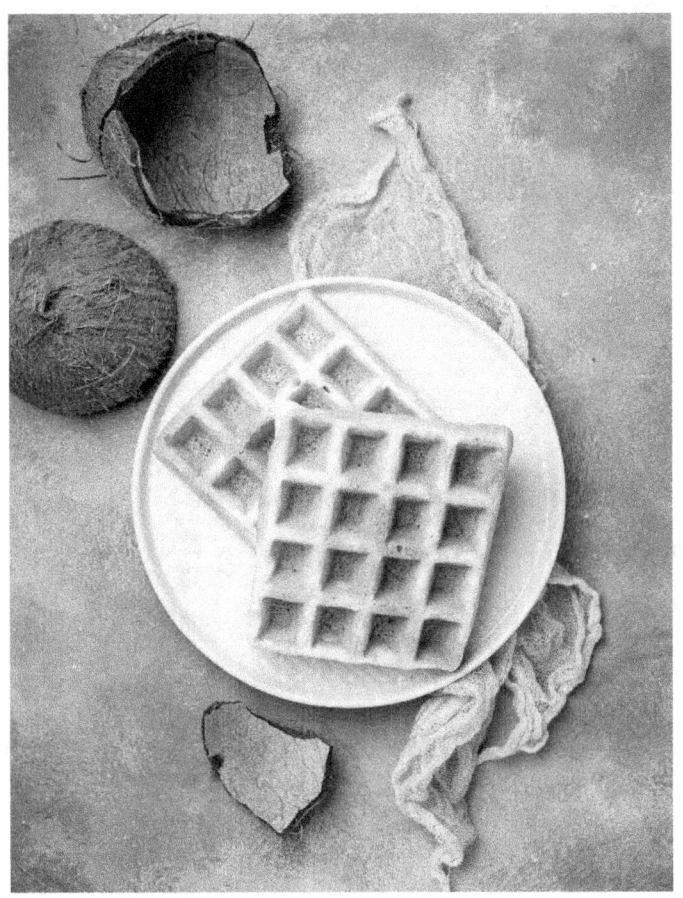

Preparation Time: 12 minutes

Cooking Time: 5 minutes

Servings: 4

Ingredients:

- 1/3 cup coconut flour
- 4 tablespoons butter, melted
- 6 organic eggs
- ½ teaspoon salt
- 1/8 teaspoon Stevia drops
- ½ teaspoon baking powder

Directions:

1. Add eggs along with butter into your blender and blend until well combined.
2. Pour egg mixture into mixing bowl. Add coconut flour, Stevia, baking powder and salt, mix well. Set aside for 5 minutes.
3. Heat your waffle iron, once it is hot pour batter and cook for 5 minutes or according to your waffle iron instructions.
4. Serve and enjoy!

Nutritional Values (Per Serving):

Calories: 247 Fat: 19 g Carbohydrates: 6 g Sugar: 1 g Protein: 11 g Cholesterol: 309 mg

Vanilla Chia Breakfast Pudding

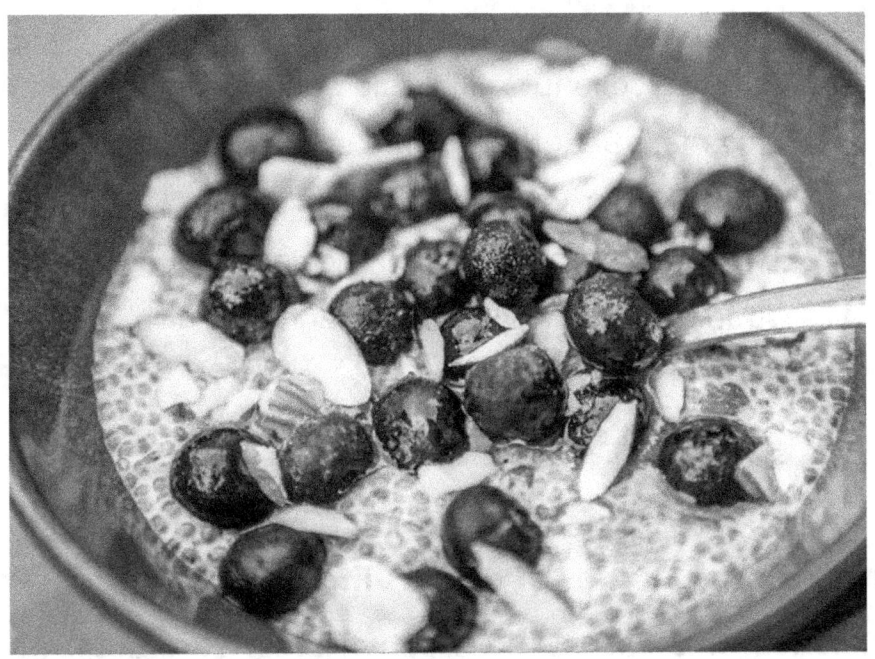

Preparation Time: 10 minutes

Servings: 2

Ingredients:

- ½ cup blueberries for topping
- 2 cups coconut milk, unsweetened
- 6 tablespoons chia seeds

- ½ teaspoon vanilla extract

Directions:

1. Add the coconut milk, chia seeds, vanilla to a glass jar. Seal the jar and shake well.
2. Place the jar in the fridge overnight.
3. The next morning pour the chia breakfast pudding into serving bowls and top with blueberries.
4. Serve and enjoy!

Nutritional Values (Per Serving):

Calories: 223 Fat: 12 g Carbohydrates: 18 g Sugar: 2 g Protein: 10 g Cholesterol: 0 mg

Classic French Toasts

Preparation Time: 10 minutes

Cooking Time: 6 minutes

Serving: 6 minutes

Ingredients:

For the glass dish bread:
- 2 tbsp flax seed meal + 6 tbsp water
- 2 tbsp coconut flour
- 2 tbsp almond flour
- 1 tsp butter
- 1½ tsp baking powder
- A pinch salt
- 2 tbsp coconut cream

For the toast's batter:
- 2 tbsp coconut milk
- 2 tbsp flax seed meal + 6 tbsp water
- ½ tsp cinnamon powder + extra for garnishing
- 1 pinch salt
- 2 tbsp butter

Directions:

For the glass dish bread:

1. For the flax egg, whisk both quantities of flax seed powder with mixing water in two separate bowls and leave to soak for 5 minutes.
2. Then, grease a glass dish (for the microwave) with the butter.
3. In another bowl, mix the coconut flour, almond flour, baking powder, and salt.
4. When the flax seed egg is ready, whisk one portion with the coconut cream and add the mixture to the dry ingredients. Continue whisking until the mixture is smooth with no lumps.
5. Pour the dough into the glass dish and microwave for 2 minutes or until the middle part of the bread is done.
6. Take out and allow the bread to cool. Then, remove the bread and slice in half. Return to the glass dish.

For the toast:

7. Whisk the mixture the remaining flax egg with the coconut cream, cinnamon powder, and salt until well combined.
8. Pour the mixture over the bread slices and leave to soak. Turn the bread a few times to soak in as much of the batter.
9. Next, melt the butter in a frying pan and fry the bread slices in the butter on both sides.
10. When golden brown on both sides, transfer the bread to a serving plate, sprinkle with cinnamon powder, and serve immediately with a cup of tea or bulletproof coffee.

Nutrition:

Calories: 96, Total Fat: 9.9g, Saturated Fat: 6.7g, Total Carbs: 2g, Dietary Fiber: 1g, Sugar: 1g, Protein: 1g, Sodium: 66mg

Avocado and Kale Soup

Preparation time: 5 minutes

Cooking time: 7 minutes

Servings: 4

Ingredients:

- 4 cups kale, torn
- 1 teaspoon turmeric powder
- Juice of 1 lime
- 1 avocado, pitted, peeled and sliced
- 4 cups vegetable stock
- 2 garlic cloves, minced
- 1 tablespoon chives, chopped
- Salt and black pepper to the taste

Directions:

1. In a pot, combine the kale with the avocado and the other ingredients, bring to a simmer, cook over medium heat for 7 minutes, blend using an immersion blender, divide into bowls and serve.

Nutrition:

calories 234, fat 12, fiber 4, carbs 7, protein 12

Minty Arugula Soup

Preparation time: 5 minutes

Cooking time: 10 minutes

Servings: 4

Ingredients:

- 3 scallions, chopped
- 1 tablespoon olive oil
- ½ cup coconut milk
- 2 cups baby arugula
- 2 tablespoons mint, chopped
- 6 cups vegetable stock
- 2 tablespoons chives, chopped
- Salt and black pepper to the taste

Directions:

1. Heat up a pot with the oil over medium-high heat, add the scallions and sauté for 2 minutes.
2. Add the rest of the ingredients, toss, bring to a simmer and cook over medium heat for 8 minutes more.
3. Divide the soup into bowls and serve.

Nutrition:

calories 200, fat 4, fiber 2, carbs 6, protein 10

Grapes, Avocado and Spinach Salad

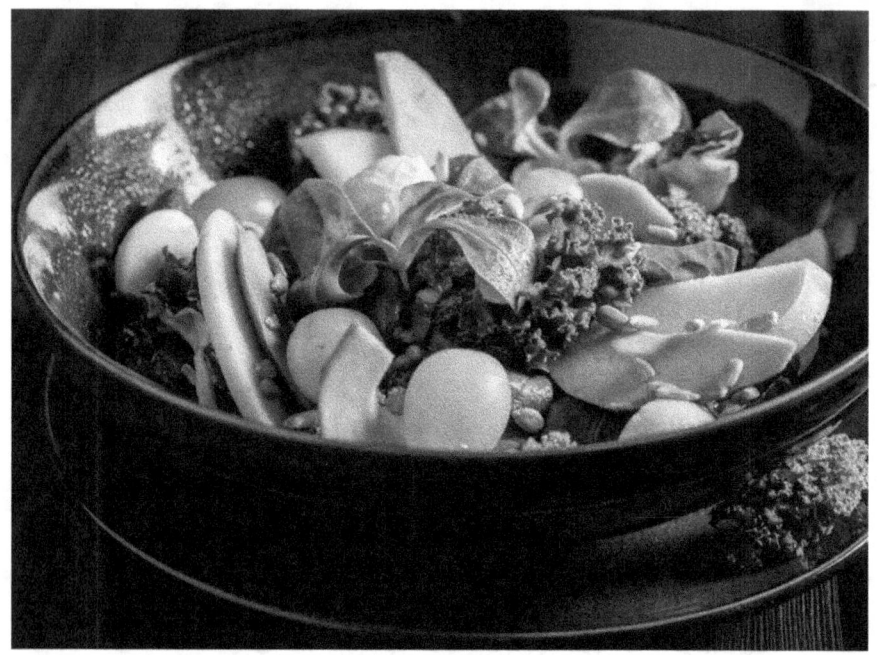

Preparation time: 10 minutes

Cooking time: 0 minutes

Servings: 4

Ingredients:

- 2 cups baby spinach
- 1 cup green grapes, halved

- 1 avocado, pitted, peeled and cubed
- 2 tablespoons olive oil
- 1 tablespoon thyme, chopped
- 1 tablespoon rosemary, chopped
- Salt and black pepper to the taste
- 1 tablespoon lime juice
- 1 garlic clove, minced

Directions:

1. In a salad bowl, combine the grapes with the spinach and the other ingredients, toss, and serve for lunch.

Nutrition:

calories 190, fat 17.1, fiber 4.6, carbs 10.9, protein 1.7

Vinegar Cucumber, Olives and Shallots Salad

Preparation time: 10 minutes

Cooking time: 0 minutes

Servings: 4

Ingredients:

- 1 pound cucumbers, sliced
- ¼ cup balsamic vinegar
- 1 cup black olives, pitted and sliced
- 3 tablespoons shallots, chopped
- 1 tablespoon dill, chopped
- A pinch of salt and black pepper
- 3 tablespoons avocado oil

Directions:

1. In a bowl, mix the cucumbers with the olives, shallots and the other ingredients, toss well, divide between plates and serve.

Nutrition:

calories 120, fat 3, fiber 2, carbs 5, protein 10

Parsley Chard Salad

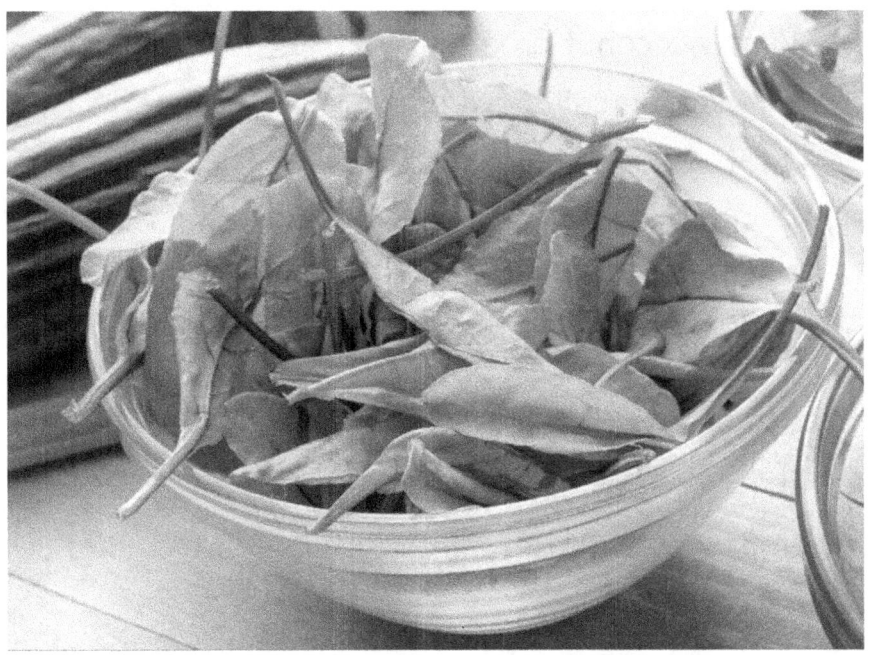

Preparation time: 10 minutes

Cooking time: 0 minutes

Servings: 4

Ingredients:

- 1 pound red chard, steamed and torn
- 1 cup grapes, halved

- 1 celery stalk, chopped
- 1 cup cherry tomatoes, halved
- 3 tablespoons balsamic vinegar
- ½ cup coconut cream
- 1 teaspoon chili powder
- 2 tablespoons olive oil
- ½ cup parsley, minced
- A pinch of sea salt and black pepper

Directions:

1. In a bowl, combine the chard with the grapes, tomatoes and the other ingredients, toss and serve right away.

Nutrition:

calories 250, fat 4, fiber 8, carbs 20, protein 6.5

Avocado, Endive and Asparagus Mix

Preparation time: 10 minutes

Cooking time: 10 minutes

Servings: 4

Ingredients:

- 2 endives, shredded
- 4 asparagus spears, trimmed and halved
- 2 avocados, peeled, pitted and sliced
- 2 tablespoons sesame seeds
- 2 tablespoons avocado oil
- A pinch of sea salt and black pepper
- Juice of 1 lime
- Black pepper to the taste
- 1 tablespoon chives, chopped

Directions:

1. Heat up a pan with the oil over medium heat, add the endives, asparagus, avocados and the other ingredients, toss, cook for 10 minutes, divide between plates and serve.

Nutrition:

calories 111, fat 2, fiber 5, carbs 8, protein 2

Keto Taco Skillet

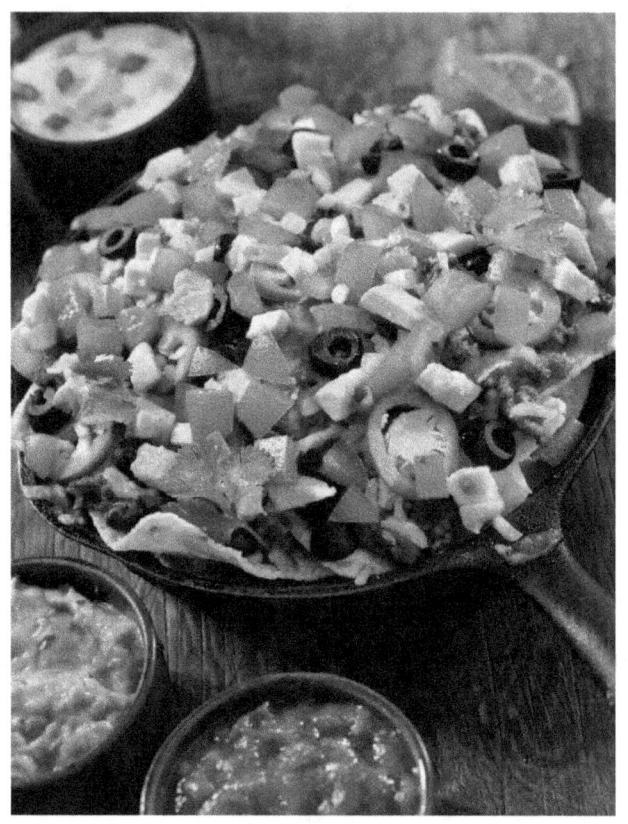

Preparation Time: 10 minutes

Cooking Time: 5 minutes

Serves: 4

Ingredients:

- 2 Tomatoes, diced
- 1 cup Textured Vegetable Protein
- 1 packet Taco Seasoning Mix
- 1 Bell Pepper, sliced into strips
- 3 cups Baby Spinach
- 2 tbsp Avocado Oil

Directions:

1. Stir together TVP and taco seasoning mix in a bowl. Pour in 2 cups of boiling water and leave for 10 minutes.
2. Heat avocado oil in a skillet.
3. Add seasoned TVP and stir for 2-3 minutes.
4. Stir in baby spinach for another minute or until slightly wilted.
5. Season to taste with salt and pepper as needed.

Nutritional Values:

Kcal per serve: 171 Fat: 11 g. Protein: 10 g. Carbs: 9 g.

Vietnamese "Vermicelli" Salad

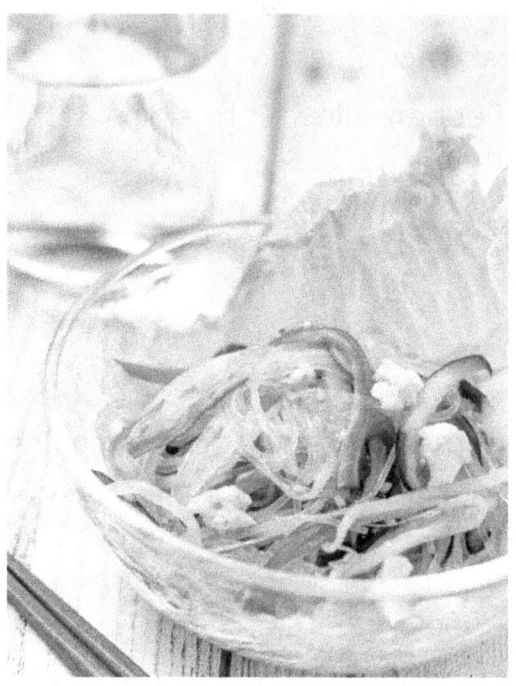

Preparation Time: 5 min

Cooking Time: Serves: 4

Ingredients:

- 100 grams Carrot, sliced into thin strips
- 2 tbsp Roasted Peanuts, roughly chopped
- 200 grams Cucumbers, spiralized
- ¼ cup Fresh Mint, chopped

- ¼ cup Fresh Cilantro, chopped
- tbsp Vegan Fish Sauce
- 1 tbsp Stevia
- 2 tbsp Fresh Lime Juice
- 2 cloves Garlic, minced
- 1 Green Chili, deseeded and minced
- 2 tbsp Sesame Oil

Directions:

1. Whisk together sugar, lime juice, sesame oil, fish sauce, minced garlic, and chopped chili. Set aside.
2. In a bowl, toss together cucumbers, carrots, cucumbers, peanuts, mint, cilantro, and prepared dressing.
3. Serve chilled.

Nutritional Values:

Kcal per serve: 249 Fat: 11 g. Protein: 5 g. Carbs: 8 g.

Simple Garlic Cauliflower Couscous

Preparation Time: 30 minutes

Servings: 3

Ingredients:

- 1 medium cauliflower head, cut into florets
- 2 tsp garlic, dried
- 2 tsp parsley, dried
- Salt

Directions:

1. Add cauliflower florets into the food processor and process until it looks like couscous.
2. Heat large pan over medium-low heat.
3. Add cauliflower couscous, parsley, and garlic in the pan and cook until softened.
4. Stir well and season with salt.
5. Serve and enjoy.

Nutritional Value (Amount per Serving):

Calories 51 Fat 0.2 g Carbohydrates 10 g Sugar 4 g Protein 3 g Cholesterol 0 mg

Mushroom Curry Pie

Preparation Time: 15 minutes

Cooking Time: 55 minutes

Serving: 4

Ingredients:

For the piecrust:

- 1 tbsp flax seed powder + 3 tbsp water
- ¾ cup coconut flour
- 4 tbsp chia seeds
- 1 tbsp psyllium husk powder
- 4 tbsp almond flour
- 1 tsp baking powder
- 1 pinch salt
- 3 tbsp olive oil
- 4 tbsp water

For the filling:

- 1 cup chopped cremini mushrooms
- 1 cup vegan mayonnaise
- ½ red bell pepper, finely chopped
- 1 tsp turmeric powder
- 3 tbsp + 9 tbsp water

- ½ tsp paprika powder
- ½ tsp garlic powder
- ¼ tsp black pepper
- ½ cup cashew cream
- 1¼ cups shredded tofu cheese

Directions:

1. In two separate bowls, mix the different portions of flax seed powder with the respective quantity of water and set aside to absorb for 5 minutes.
2. Preheat the oven to 350 F.

Make the crust:

3. When the flax egg is ready, pour the smaller quantity into a food processor, add the coconut flour, chia seeds, almond flour, psyllium husk powder, baking powder, salt, olive oil, and water. Blend the ingredients until a ball forms out of the dough.
4. Line a springform pan with an 8-inch diameter parchment paper and grease the pan with cooking spray.
5. Spread the dough in the bottom of the pan and bake in the oven for 15 minutes.

Make the filling:

6. In a bowl, add the remaining flax egg, mushrooms, mayonnaise, water, bell pepper, turmeric, paprika, garlic powder, black pepper, cashew cream, and tofu cheese. Combine the mixture evenly and fill the piecrust. Bake further for 40 minutes or until the pie is golden brown.
7. Remove, slice, and serve the pie with a chilled strawberry drink.

Nutrition:

Calories:548, Total Fat: 55.9g, Saturated Fat:8.5 g, Total Carbs: 6g, Dietary Fiber:2 g, Sugar: 2g, Protein:8 g, Sodium: 405mg

Green Avocado Carbonara

Preparation Time: 15minutes

Cooking Time: 15minutes

Serving: 4

Ingredients:

- 8 tbsp flax seed powder + 1 ½ cups water
- 1 ½ cups dairy-free cashew cream
- 1 tsp salt
- 5 ½ tbsp psyllium husk powder

Avocado sauce

- 1 avocado, peeled and pitted
- 1 ¾ cups coconut cream
- Juice of ½ lemon
- ½ teaspoon garlic powder
- ¼ cup olive oil
- 1 teaspoon onion powder
- ¾ teaspoon sea salt
- ¼ teaspoon black pepper
- Walnut Parmesan or store-bought parmesan

For serving

- 4 tbsp toasted pecans
- ½ cup freshly grated tofu cheese

Directions:

1. Preheat the oven to 300 F.
2. In a medium bowl, mix the flax seed powder with water and allow sitting to thicken for 5 minutes.
3. Add the cashew cream, salt, and psyllium husk powder. Whisk until smooth batter forms.
4. Line a baking sheet with parchment paper, pour in the batter and cover with another parchment paper. Use a rolling pin to flatten the dough into the sheet.
5. Place in the oven and bake for 10 to 12 minutes. Remove the pasta after, take off the parchment papers and use a sharp knife to slice the pasta into thin strips lengthwise. Cut each piece into halves, pour into a bowl, and set aside.
6. For the avocado sauce, in a blender, combine the avocado, coconut cream, lemon juice, onion powder, and garlic powder. Puree the Ingredients until smooth.

7. Pour the olive oil over the pasta and stir to coat properly. Pour the avocado sauce on top and mix. Then, season with salt, black pepper, and the soy cheese. Combine again.
8. Divide the pasta into serving plates, garnish with extra soy cheese and pecans, and serve immediately.

Nutrition:

Calories:941, Total Fat:94.2g, Saturated Fat:30.4g, Total Carbs:19g, Dietary Fiber:8g, Sugar:5g, Protein:16g, Sodium:1314mg

Herbed Zucchinis and Olives

Preparation time: 10 minutes

Cooking time: 20 minutes

Servings: 4

Ingredients:

- 1 cup kalamata olives, pitted
- 1 cup green olives, pitted
- 1 pound zucchinis, roughly cubed
- 1 tablespoon basil, chopped
- 1 tablespoon rosemary, chopped
- 1 tablespoon cilantro, chopped
- 2 tablespoons olive oil
- 3 garlic cloves, minced
- 1 tablespoon lemon juice
- 1 teaspoon lemon zest, grated
- 1 tablespoon sweet paprika
- A pinch of salt and black pepper

Directions:

1. Heat up a pan with the oil over medium heat, add the garlic, lemon zest and paprika and sauté for 2 minutes.
2. Add the olives, zucchinis and the other ingredients, toss, cook over medium heat for 18 minutes more, divide between plates and serve.

Nutrition:

calories 200, fat 20, fiber 4, carbs 3, protein 1

Veggie Pan

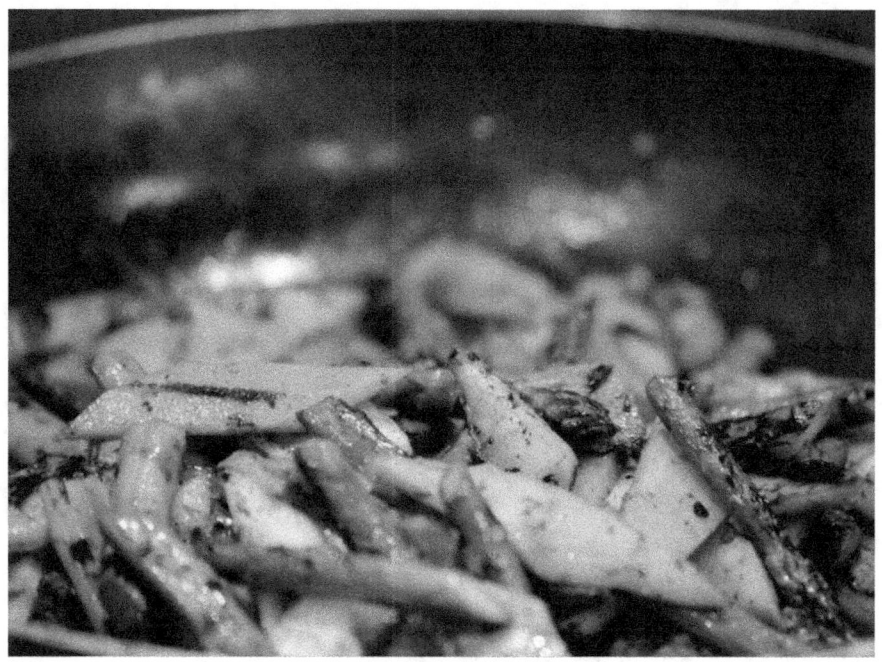

Preparation time: 10 minutes

Cooking time: 20 minutes

Servings: 4

Ingredients:

- 1 cup green beans, trimmed and halved
- 1 cup cherry tomatoes, halved
- 1 eggplant, cubed

- 1 red bell pepper, cut into strips
- 1 zucchini, roughly cubed
- 3 scallions, chopped
- 2 tablespoons olive oil
- 2 tablespoons lime juice
- Salt and black pepper to the taste
- 1 teaspoon chili powder
- 1 tablespoon cilantro, chopped
- 3 garlic cloves, minced

Directions:

1. Heat up a pan with the oil over medium heat, add the scallions, chili powder and the garlic and sauté for 5 minutes.
2. Add the green beans, tomatoes and the other ingredients, toss, cook over medium heat for 15 minutes.
3. Divide the mix between plates and serve as a side dish.

Nutrition:

calories 137, fat 7.7, fiber 7.1, carbs 18.1, protein 3.4

Beet and Cabbage

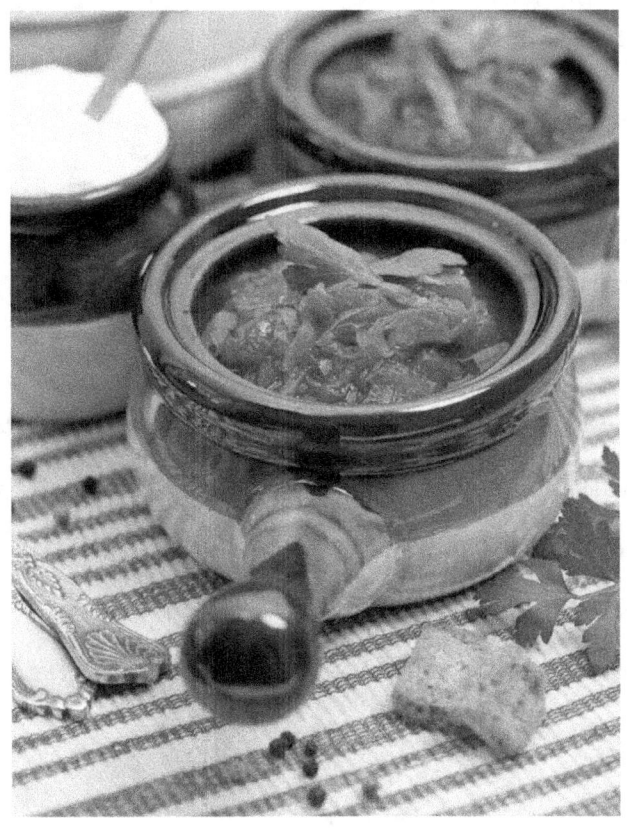

Preparation time: 10 minutes

Cooking time: 20 minutes

Servings: 4

Ingredients:

- 1 green cabbage head, shredded
- 1 yellow onion, chopped
- 1 beet, peeled and cubed
- 2 tablespoons olive oil
- ½ cup chicken stock
- A pinch of salt and black pepper
- 2 tablespoons chives, chopped

Directions:

1. Heat up a pan with the oil over medium heat, add the onion and sauté for 5 minutes.
2. Add the cabbage and the other ingredients, toss, cook over medium heat for 15 minutes more, divide between plates and serve.

Nutrition:

calories 128, fat 7.3, fiber 5.6, carbs 15.6, protein 3.1

Broccoli with Brussels Sprouts

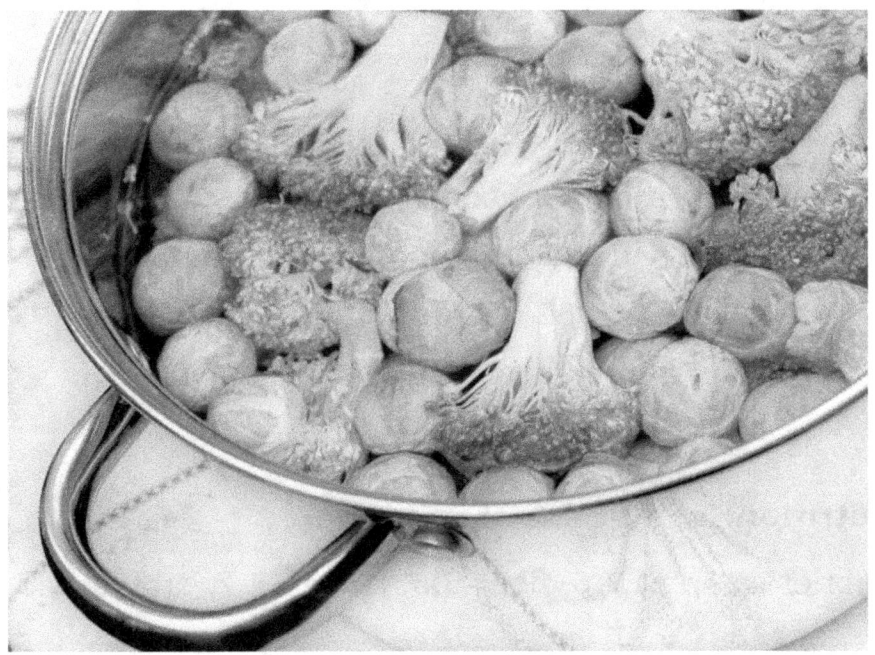

Preparation time: 10 minutes

Cooking time: 25 minutes

Servings: 4

Ingredients:

- 1 pound broccoli florets
- ½ pound Brussels sprouts, trimmed and halved
- 1 tablespoon ginger, grated

- 2 tablespoons olive oil
- 1 tablespoon balsamic vinegar
- A pinch of salt and black pepper

Directions:

1. In a roasting pan, combine the broccoli with the sprouts and the other ingredients, toss gently and bake at 380 degrees F for 25 minutes.
2. Divide the mix between plates and serve.

Nutrition:

calories 129, fat 7.6, fiber 5.3, carbs 13.7, protein 5.2

Tomato Salad

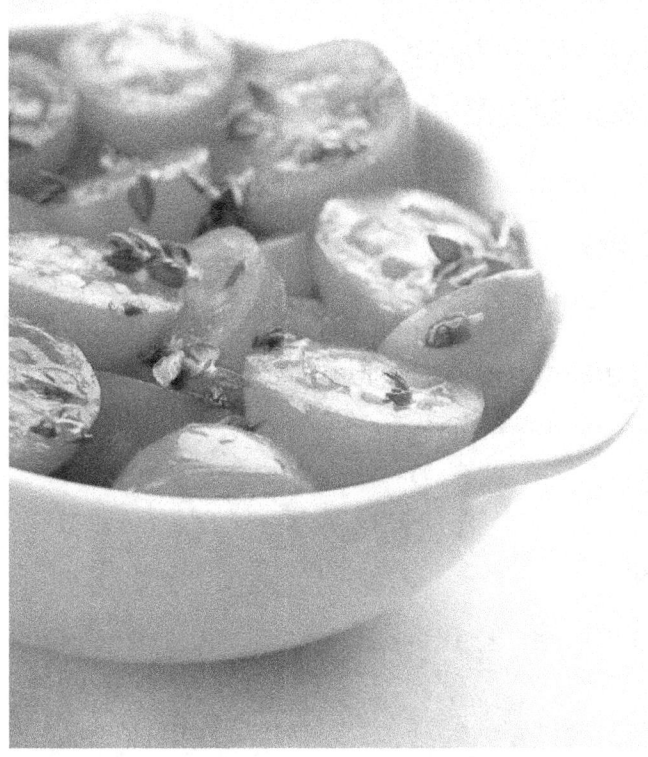

Preparation time: 10 minutes

Cooking time: 0 minutes

Servings: 4

Ingredients:

- 1 pound cherry tomatoes, halved
- 1 tablespoon olive oil
- 3 scallions, chopped
- A pinch of salt and black pepper
- 1 tablespoon lime juice
- ¼ cup parsley, chopped

Directions:

1. In a bowl, combine the tomatoes with the scallions and the other ingredients, toss and serve as a side salad.

Nutrition:

calories 180, fat 2, fiber 2, carbs 8, protein 6

Cinnamon-Scented Quinoa

Preparation Time: 5 mins

Servings: 4

Ingredients:

- Chopped walnuts
- 1 ½ c. water
- 2 cinnamon sticks
- Maple syrup
- 1 c. quinoa

Directions:

1. Add the quinoa to a bowl and wash it in several changes of water until the water is clear. When washing quinoa, rub grains and allow them to settle before you pour off the water.
2. Use a large fine-mesh sieve to drain the quinoa. Prepare your pressure cooker with a trivet and steaming basket. Place the quinoa and the cinnamon sticks in the basket and pour the water.

3. Close and lock the lid. Cook at high pressure for 6 minutes. When the cooking time is up, release the pressure using the quick release method.
4. Fluff the quinoa with a fork and remove the cinnamon sticks. Divide the cooked quinoa among serving bowls and top with maple syrup and chopped walnuts.

Nutrition:

Calories: 160, Fat:3 g, Carbs:28 g, Protein:6 g, Sugars:19 g, Sodium:40 mg

Spinach and Kale Mix

Preparation Time: 5 mins

Servings: 4

Ingredients:

- 2 chopped shallots
- 2 c. baby spinach
- 1 c. no-salt-added and chopped canned tomatoes
- 2 minced garlic cloves
- 5 c. torn kale
- 1 tbsp. olive oil

Directions:

1. Heat up a pan with the oil over medium-high heat, add the shallots, stir and sauté for 5 minutes.
2. Add the spinach, kale and the other ingredients, toss, cook for 10 minutes more, divide between plates and serve.

Nutrition:

Calories: 89, Fat:3.7 g, Carbs:12.4 g, Protein:3.6 g, Sugars:0 g, Sodium:50 mg

Celery Soup

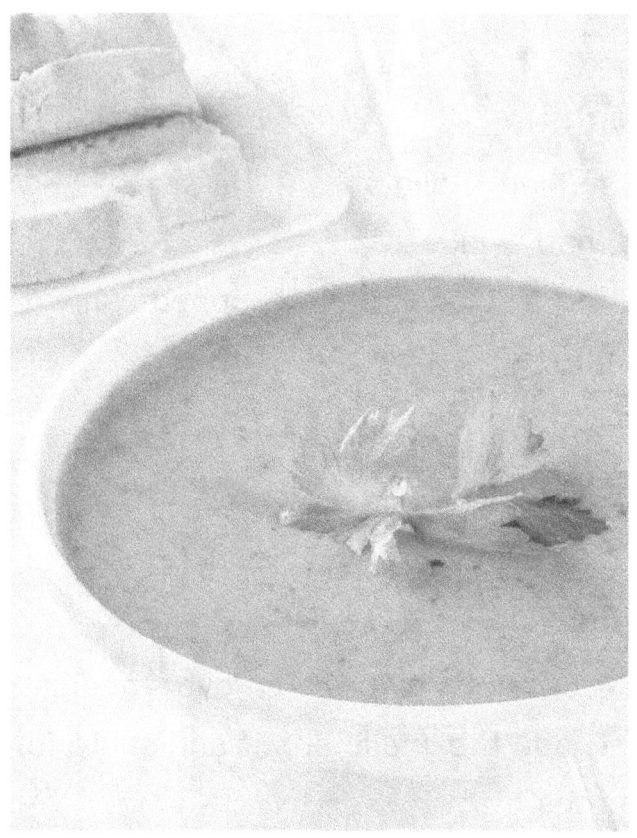

Preparation time: 10 minutes

Cooking time: 25 minutes

Servings: 8

Ingredients:

- 26 ounces celery leaves, and stalks, chopped
- 1 tablespoon dried onion flakes
- 3 teaspoons fenugreek powder
- 3 teaspoons vegetable stock powder
- Salt and ground black pepper, to taste
- 10 ounces sour cream

Directions:

1. Put the celery into a pot, add the water to cover, add the onion flakes, salt, pepper, stock powder, and fenugreek powder, stir, bring to a boil over medium heat, and simmer for 20 minutes.
2. Use an immersion blender to make the cream, add the sour cream, more salt and pepper, and blend again.
3. Heat up soup again over medium heat, ladle into bowls, and serve.

Nutrition:

Calories - 140, Fat - 2, Fiber - 1, Carbs - 5, Protein - 10

Spinach Soup

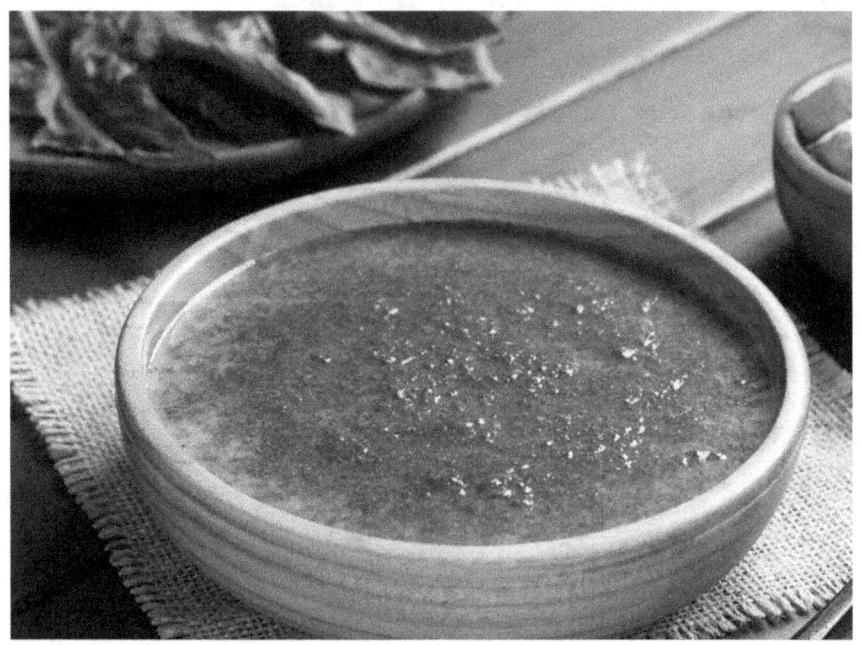

Preparation time: 10 minutes

Cooking time: 15 minutes

Servings: 8

Ingredients:

- 20 ounces spinach, chopped
- 2 tablespoons butter
- 1 teaspoon garlic, minced

- 45 ounces chicken stock
- ½ teaspoon ground nutmeg
- Salt and ground black pepper, to taste
- 2 cups heavy cream
- 1 onion, peeled and chopped

Directions:

1. Heat up a pot with the butter over medium heat, add the onion, stir, and cook for 4 minutes.
2. Add the garlic, stir, and cook for 1 minute.
3. Add the spinach and stock, stir, and cook for 5 minutes.
4. Blend soup with an immersion blender, and heat up the soup again.
5. Add the salt, pepper, nutmeg, and cream, stir, and cook for 5 minutes.
6. Ladle into bowls and serve.

Nutrition:

Calories - 245, Fat - 24, Fiber - 3, Carbs - 4, Protein - 6

Alfalfa Sprouts Salad

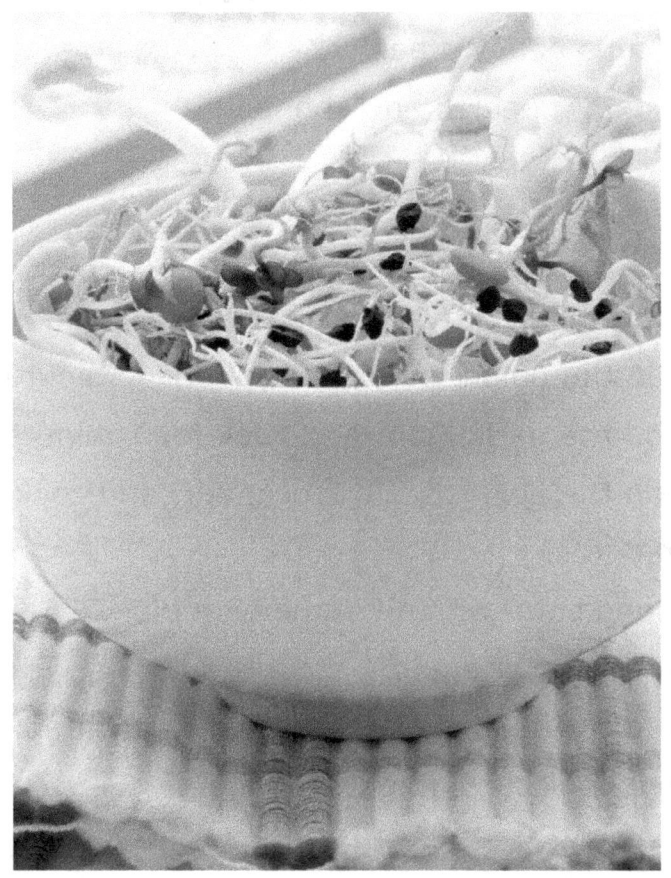

Preparation time: 10 minutes

Cooking time: 0 minutes

Servings: 4

Ingredients:

- 1 green apple, cored, and julienned
- 1½ teaspoons dark sesame oil
- 4 cups alfalfa sprouts
- 1½ teaspoons grape seed oil
- ¼ cup coconut milk yogurt
- 4 nasturtium leaves
- Salt and ground black pepper, to taste

Directions:

1. In a salad bowl, mix the sprouts with apple and nasturtium.
2. Add the salt, pepper, sesame oil, grape seed oil, and coconut yogurt, toss to coat, and divide on plates, and serve.

Nutrition:

Calories - 100, Fat - 3, Fiber - 1, Carbs - 2, Protein - 6

Fried Okra

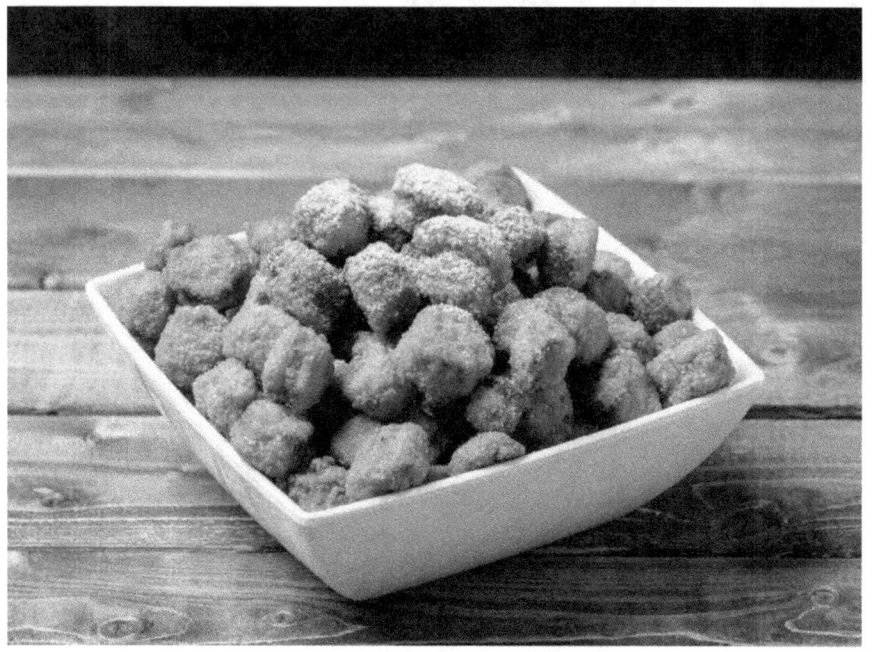

Preparation Time: 10 minutes

Cooking Time: 10 minutes

Servings: 4

Ingredients:

- 1 lb fresh okra, cut into ¼" slices
- 1/3 cup almond meal
- Salt

- Pepper
- Oil for frying

Directions:

1. Heat oil in large pan over medium-high heat.
2. In a bowl, mix together sliced okra, almond meal, pepper, and salt until well coated.
3. Once the oil is hot then add okra to the hot oil and cook until lightly browned.
4. Remove fried okra from pan and allow to drain on paper towels.
5. Serve and enjoy.

Nutritions:

Calories 91 Fat 4.2 g Carbohydrates 10.2 g Sugar 10.2 g Protein 3.9 g Cholesterol 0 mg

Avocado Broccoli Soup

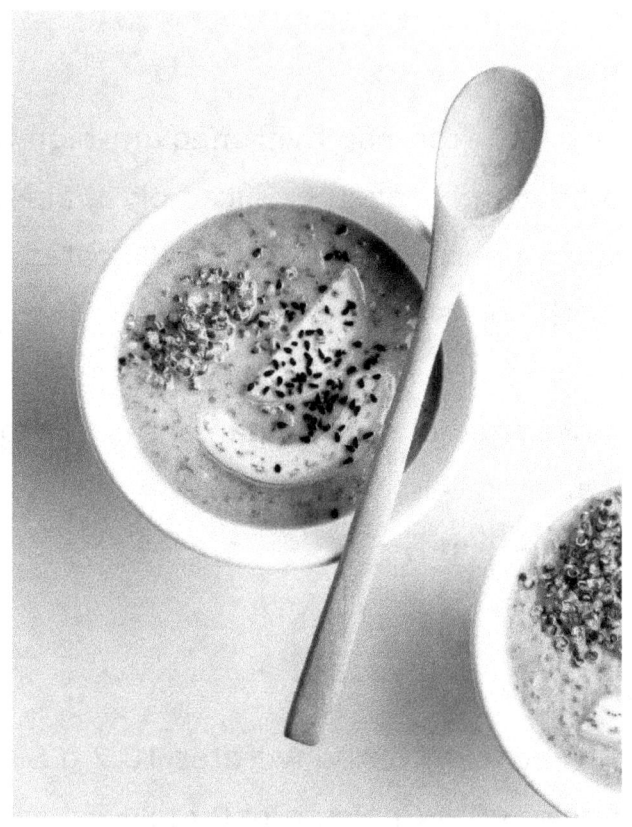

Preparation Time: 20 minutes

Cooking Time: 5 minutes

Servings: 4

Ingredients:

- 2 cups broccoli florets, chopped
- 2 avocados, chopped
- 5 cups vegetable broth
- Pepper
- Salt

Directions:

1. Cook broccoli in boiling water for 5 minutes. Drain well.
2. Add broccoli, vegetable broth, avocados, pepper, and salt to the blender and blend until smooth.
3. Stir well and serve warm.

Nutritions:

Calories 269 Fat 21.5 g Carbohydrates 12.8 g Sugar 2.1 g Protein 9.2 g Cholesterol 0 mg

Carrot Soup

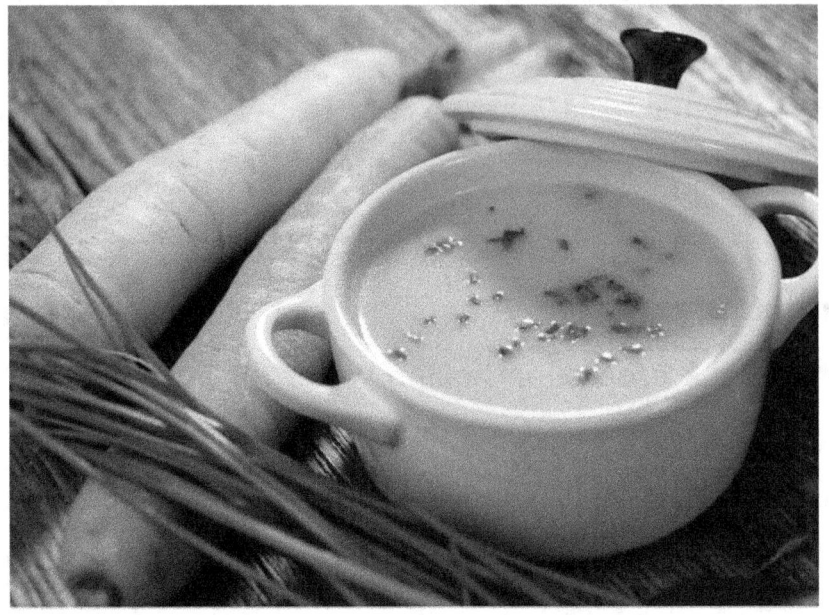

Preparation time: 10 minutes

Cooking time: 5 hours

Servings: 6

Ingredients:

- 2 potatoes, cubed
- 1 yellow onion, chopped
- 3 pounds carrots, cubed

- 1-quart veggie stock
- 1 teaspoon thyme, dried
- 3 tablespoons coconut milk
- 2 teaspoons curry powder
- Salt and black pepper to the taste
- 3 tablespoons vegan cheese, crumbled
- A handful pistachios, chopped

Directions:

1. In your slow cooker, mix onion with potatoes, carrots, stock, salt, pepper, thyme and curry powder, stir, cover, cook on High for 1 hour and on Low for 4 hours.
2. Add coconut milk, stir, blend soup using an immersion blender, ladle soup into bowls, sprinkle vegan cheese and pistachios on top and serve.
3. Enjoy!

Nutritions:

calories 241, fat 4, fiber 7, carbs 10, protein 4

Zucchini Soup

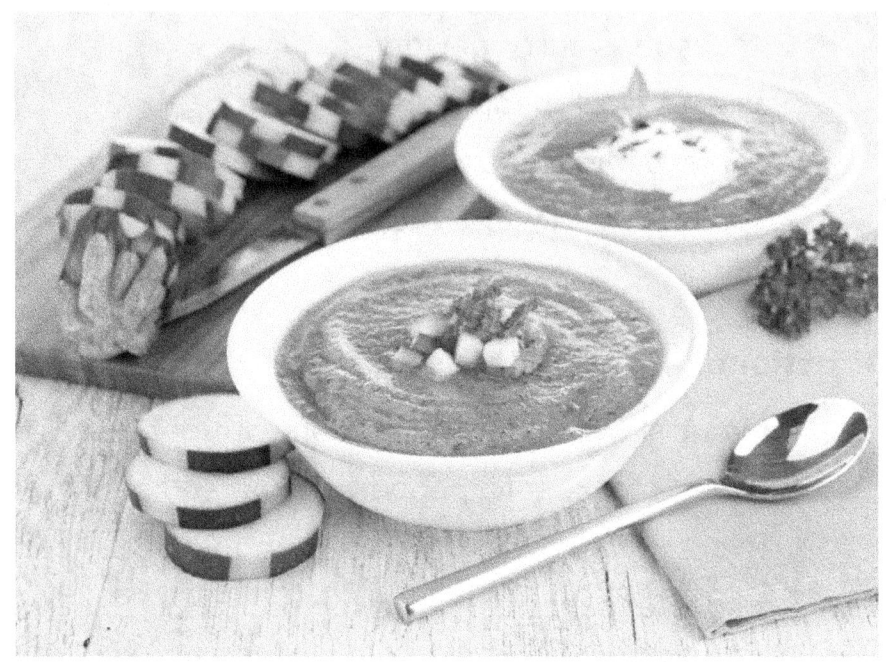

Preparation Time: 10 minutes

Cooking Time: 10 minutes

Servings: 8

Ingredients:

- 2 ½ lbs zucchini, peeled and sliced
- 4 cups vegetable stock
- 1/3 cup basil leaves

- 4 garlic cloves, chopped
- 2 tbsp olive oil
- 1 medium onion, diced
- Pepper
- Salt

Directions:

1. Heat olive oil in a pan over medium-low heat.
2. Add zucchini and onion and sauté until softened. Add garlic and sauté for a minute.
3. Add vegetable stock and simmer for 15 minutes.
4. Remove from heat. Stir in basil and puree the soup using a blender until smooth and creamy. Season with pepper and salt.
5. Stir well and serve.

Nutritions:

Calories 62, Fat 4g, Carbohydrates 6.8g, Sugar 3.3g, Protein 2g, Cholesterol 0mg

Almond Soup With Cardamom

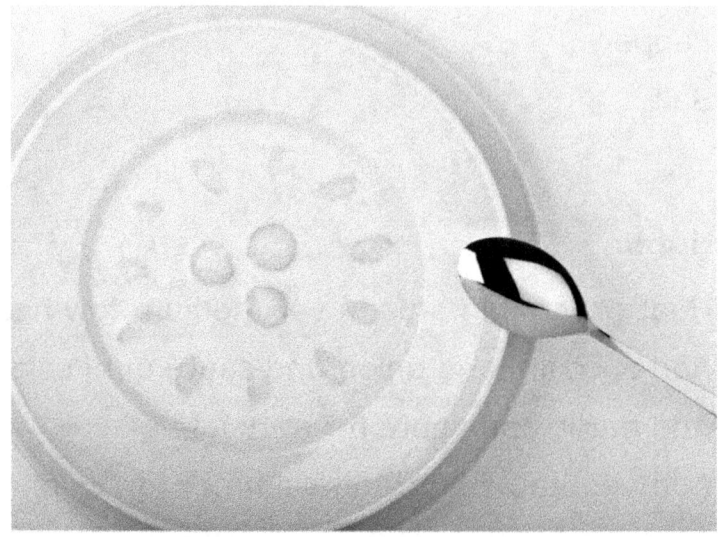

Preparation time: 5 minutes

cooking time: 35 minutes total: 40minutes

servings: 4

Ingredients

- 1 tablespoon olive oil
- 1 medium onion, chopped
- 1 medium red bell pepper, chopped
- 1 medium russet potato, chopped
- 1/2 cup almond butter

- 4 cups vegetable broth, homemade (see Light Vegetable Broth or store-bought, or water
- 1/2 teaspoon ground cardamom
- Salt and freshly ground black pepper
- 1/4 cup sliced toasted almonds, for garnish

Directions

1. In a large soup pot, heat the oil over medium heat. Add the onion, potato, and bell pepper. Cover and cook until softened, about 5 minutes. Add the broth, cardamom, and salt and pepper to taste. Bring to a boil, then reduce heat to low and simmer, uncovered, until the vegetables are tender, about 30 minutes.
2. Add the almond butter and puree in the pot with an immersion blender or in a blender or food processor, in batches if necessary, and return to the pot. Reheat over medium heat until hot. Taste, adjusting seasonings if necessary, and add more broth or some soy milk if needed for desired consistency.
3. Ladle the soup into bowls, sprinkle with toasted sliced almonds, and serve.

Squash Soup With Pecans And Ginger

Preparation time: 10 minutes

cooking time: 30 minutes

servings: 4

Ingredients

- 1/3 cup toasted pecans
- 2 tablespoons chopped crystallized ginger
- 1 celery rib, chopped
- 1 tablespoon canola or grapeseed oil
- 1 medium onion, chopped
- 1 teaspoon grated fresh ginger
- 5 cups vegetable broth, homemade (see Light Vegetable Broth or store-bought, or water
- 1 kabocha squash, peeled, seeded, and cut into 1/2-inch dice
- 1/4 cup pure maple syrup
- 2 tablespoons soy sauce
- 1/4 teaspoon ground allspice
- Salt and freshly ground black pepper
- 1 cup plain unsweetened soy milk

Directions

1. In a food processor, combine the pecans and crystallized ginger and pulse until coarsely chopped. Set aside.
2. In a large soup pot, heat the oil over medium heat. Add the onion, celery, and fresh ginger. Cover and cook until softened, about 5 minutes. Stir in the broth and squash, cover, and bring to a boil. Reduce the heat to low and simmer, covered, occasionally stirring, until the squash is tender, about 30 minutes.
3. Stir in the maple syrup, soy sauce, allspice, and salt and pepper to taste. Puree in the pot with an immersion blender or in a blender or food processor, in batches if necessary, and return to the pot.
4. Stir in the soy milk and heat over low heat until hot. Ladle the soup into bowls and sprinkle with the pecan and ginger mixture, and serve.

Balsamic Lentil Stew

Preparation time: 10 minutes

cooking time: 30 minutes

servings: 5

Ingredients

- 1 onion, chopped
- 1 teaspoon olive oil
- 4 carrots, peeled and chopped
- 3 garlic cloves, minced
- 2 tablespoons balsamic vinegar
- 4 cups Economical Vegetable Broth or water
- 1 (28-ouncecan crushed tomatoes
- 2 cups dried lentils or 2 (15-ouncecans lentils, drained and rinsed
- 1 tablespoon sugar
- 1 teaspoon salt
- Freshly ground black pepper

Directions

1. Preparing the Ingredients
2. Heat the olive oil in a large soup pot over

medium heat.

3. Add the carrots, onion, and garlic and sauté for about 5 minutes, until the vegetables are softened. Pour in the vinegar, and let it sizzle to deglaze the bottom of the pot. Add the vegetable broth, tomatoes, sugar, and lentils.
4. Bring to a boil, then reduce the heat to low. Simmer for about 25 minutes, until the lentils are soft. Add the salt and season to taste with pepper. Leftovers will keep in an airtight container for up to 1 week in the refrigerator or up to 1 month in the freezer.

Nutrition (2 cups)

Calories: 353; Protein: 22g; Total fat: 2g; Saturated fat: 0g; Carbohydrates: 67g; Fiber: 27g

Pumpkin-Pear Soup

Preparation Time: 10 Minutes

Cooking Time: 15 Minutes

Servings: 4

Ingredients

- 1 teaspoon olive oil or coconut oil
- 1 onion, diced, or 2 teaspoons onion powder
- 1-inch piece fresh ginger, peeled and diced, or 1 teaspoon ground ginger
- 1 pear, cored and chopped
- Optional spices to take the taste up a notch:
- 1 teaspoon curry powder
- ½ teaspoon pumpkin pie spice
- ½ teaspoon smoked paprika
- Pinch red pepper flakes
- 4 cups water or Economical Vegetable Broth
- 3 cups canned pumpkin purée
- 1 to 2 teaspoons salt (less if using salted broth)
- Pinch freshly ground black pepper
- ¼ to ½ cup canned coconut milk (optional)
- 2 to 4 tablespoons nutritional yeast (optional)

Directions

1. Preparing the Ingredients.
2. Heat the olive oil in a large pot over medium heat. Add the onion, ginger, and pear and sauté for about 5 minutes, until soft. Sprinkle in any optional spices and stir to combine.
3. Add the water, pumpkin, salt, and pepper, and stir until smooth and combined. Cook until just bubbling, about 10 minutes.
4. Stir in the coconut milk (if using) and nutritional yeast (if using), and remove the soup from the heat. Leftovers will keep in an airtight container for up to 1 week in the refrigerator or up to 1 month in the freezer.

Per Serving (2 cups)

Calories: 90; Protein: 2g; Total fat: 1g; Saturated fat: 0g; Carbohydrates: 17g; Fiber: 3g

Spicy Pinto Bean Soup

Preparation Time: 5 Minutes

Cooking Time: 25 Minutes

Servings: 4

Ingredients

- 4 1/2 cups cooked or 3 (15.5-ounce) cans pinto beans, drained and rinsed
- 1 (14.5-ounce) can crushed tomatoes
- 1 teaspoon chipotle chile in adobo
- 1 medium onion, chopped
- 2 tablespoons olive oil
- 1/4 cup chopped celery
- 2 garlic cloves, minced
- 1/2 teaspoon ground cumin
- 1/2 teaspoon dried oregano
- 4 cups vegetable broth, homemade (see Light Vegetable Broth) or store-bought, or water
- Salt and freshly ground black pepper
- 2 tablespoons chopped fresh cilantro, for garnish

Directions

1. In a food processor, puree 1 1/2 cups of the pinto beans with the tomatoes and chipotle. Set aside.
2. In a large soup pot, heat the oil over medium heat. Add the onion, celery, and garlic. Cover and cook until soft, occasionally stirring, about 10 minutes. Stir in the cumin, oregano, broth, pureed bean mixture, and the remaining 3 cups beans. Season with salt and pepper to taste.
3. Bring to a boil and reduce heat to low and simmer, uncovered, stirring occasionally, until the flavors are incorporated and the soup is hot, about 15 minutes. Ladle into bowls, garnish with cilantro, and serve.

Puttanesca Seitan And Spinach Salad

Preparation time: 5 minutes

cooking time: 6 minutes

servings: 4

Ingredients

- 4 tablespoons olive oil
- 8 ounces seitan, homemade or store-bought, cut into 1/2-inch strips
- 2 tablespoons capers
- 3 garlic cloves, minced
- 1/2 cup kalamata olives, pitted and halved
- 1/2 cup green olives, pitted and halved
- 3 cups fresh baby spinach, cut into strips
- 11/2 cups ripe cherry tomatoes, halved
- 2 tablespoons balsamic vinegar
- 1/4 teaspoon salt (optional)
- 1/4 teaspoon freshly ground black pepper
- 2 tablespoons torn fresh basil leaves
- 2 tablespoons minced fresh parsley

Directions

1. In a large skillet, heat 1 tablespoon of the oil over medium heat. Add the seitan and cook until browned on both sides, about 5 minutes. Add the garlic and cook until fragrant, about 30 seconds. Transfer to a large bowl and set aside to cool, about 15 minutes.
2. When the seitan has cooled to room temperature, add the kalamata and green olives, capers, spinach, and tomatoes. Set aside.
3. In a small bowl, combine the remaining 3 tablespoons oil with the vinegar, salt, and pepper. Whisk until blended, then pour the dressing over the salad. Add the basil and parsley, toss gently to combine, and serve.

Carrot And Orange Salad With Cashews And Cilantro

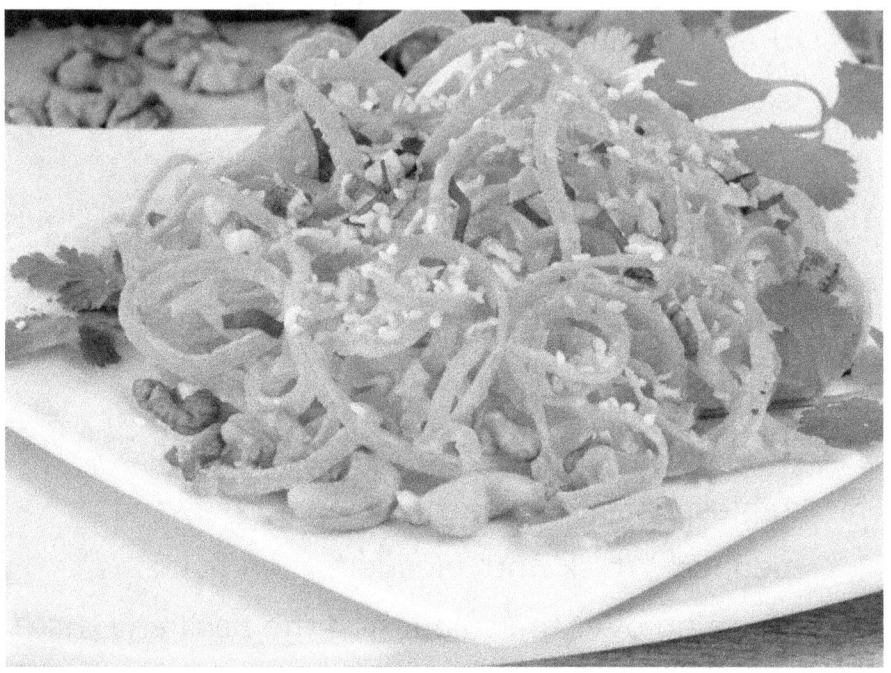

Preparation time: 15 minutes

cooking time: 0 minutes

servings: 4

Ingredients

- 1 pound carrots, shredded
- 2 oranges, peeled, segmented, and chopped
- 1/2 cup unsalted roasted cashews
- 2 tablespoons fresh lime juice
- 1/4 cup chopped fresh cilantro
- 2 tablespoons fresh orange juice
- 2 teaspoons brown sugar (optional
- Salt (optional) and freshly ground black pepper
- 1/3 cup olive oil

Directions

1. In a large bowl, combine the carrots, oranges, cashews, and cilantro and set aside.
2. In a small bowl, combine the orange juice, lime juice, sugar, and salt and pepper to taste. Whisk in the oil until blended. Pour the dressing over the carrot mixture, stirring to lightly coat. Taste, adjusting seasonings if necessary. Toss gently to combine and serve.

Dazzling Vegetable Salad

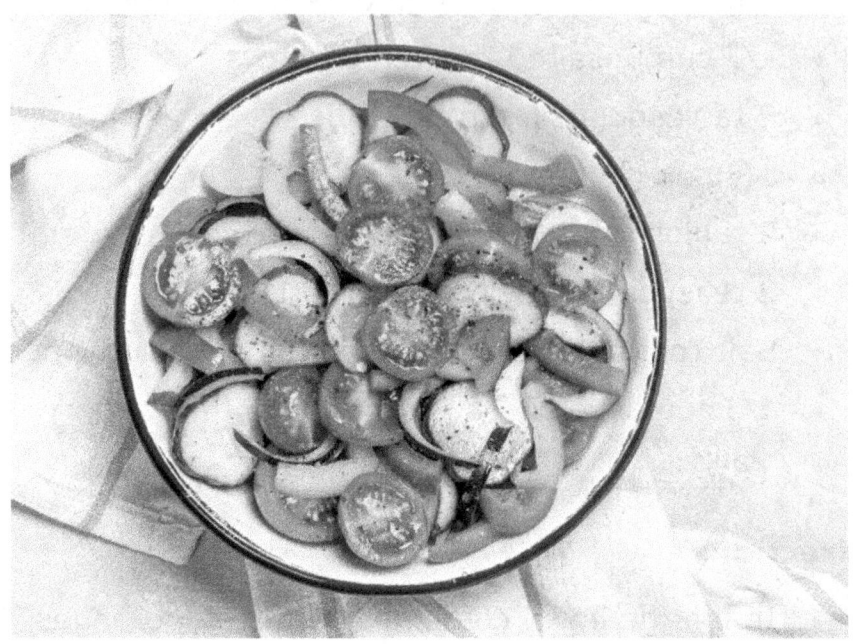

Preparation time: 15 minutes

cooking time: 0 minutes

servings: 4

Ingredients

- 1 medium carrot, shredded
- 1 cup finely shredded red cabbage
- 1 cup ripe grape or cherry tomatoes, halved

- 1 1/2 cups cooked or 1 (15.5-ounce can chickpeas, rinsed and drained
- 1 medium yellow bell pepper, cut into matchsticks
- 1/4 cup halved pitted kalamata olives
- 1 ripe Hass avocado, pitted, peeled, and cut into 1/2-inch dice
- 1/4 cup olive oil
- 1 1/2 tablespoons fresh lemon juice
- 1/2 teaspoon salt
- 1/8 teaspoon freshly ground black pepper
- Pinch sugar (optional

Directions

1. In a large bowl, combine the watercress, carrot, cabbage, tomatoes, bell pepper, chickpeas, olives, and avocado and set aside.
2. In a small bowl, combine the oil, lemon juice, salt, black pepper, and sugar. Blend well and add to the salad. Toss gently to combine and serve.

Indonesian Green BeanSalad With Cabbage And Carrots

Preparation time: 15 minutes

cooking time: 0 minutes

servings: 4

Ingredients

- 2 cups green beans, trimmed and cut into 1-inch pieces
- 2 medium carrots, cut into 1/4-inch slices
- 2 cups finely shredded cabbage
- 1/3 cup golden raisins
- 1 medium shallot, chopped
- 1/4 cup unsalted roasted peanuts
- 1 garlic clove, minced
- 11/2 teaspoons grated fresh ginger
- 1/3 cup creamy peanut butter
- 2 tablespoons soy sauce
- 2 tablespoons fresh lemon juice
- 1 teaspoon sugar(optional)
- 1/4 teaspoon salt(optional)
- 1/8 teaspoon ground cayenne

- ¾ cup unsweetened coconut milk

Directions

1. Lightly steam the green beans, carrots, and cabbage for about 5 minutes, then place them in a large bowl. Add the raisins and peanuts and set aside to cool.
2. In a food processor or blender, puree the garlic, shallot, and ginger. Add the peanut butter, soy sauce, lemon juice, sugar, salt, and cayenne, and process until blended. Add the coconut milk and blend until smooth. Pour the dressing over the salad, toss gently to combine, and serve.

Red Cabbage Slaw With Black-Vinegar Dressing

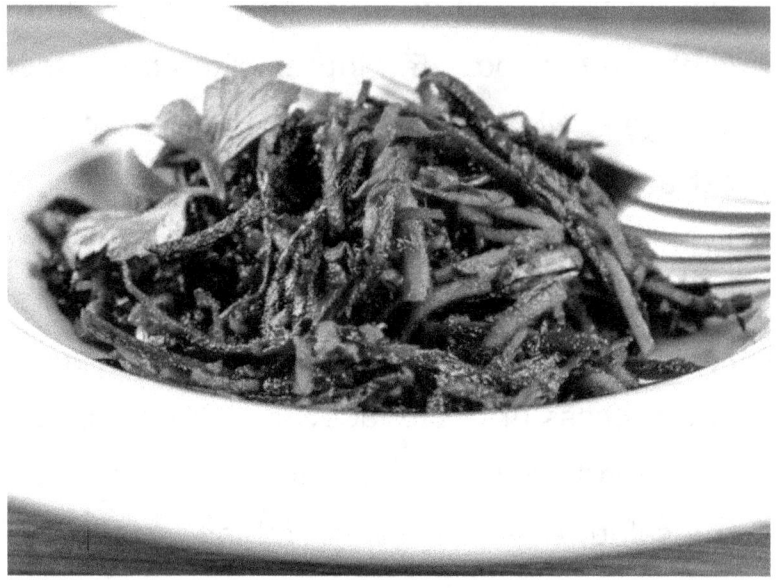

Preparation Time: 15 Minutes

Cooking Time: 0 Minutes

Servings: 6

Ingredients

- 4 cups shredded red cabbage
- 1 cup shredded daikon radish
- 2 cups thinly sliced napa cabbage

- 1/4 cup fresh orange juice
- 2 tablespoons Chinese black vinegar
- 1 tablespoon soy sauce
- 1 tablespoon toasted sesame oil
- 1 tablespoon grapeseed oil
- 1 teaspoon grated fresh ginger
- 1/2 teaspoon ground Szechuan peppercorns
- 1 tablespoon black sesame seeds, for garnish

Directions

1. In a large bowl, combine the red cabbage, napa, and daikon and set aside.
2. In a small bowl, combine the orange juice, vinegar, soy sauce, grapeseed oil, sesame oil, ginger, and peppercorns. Blend well. Pour the dressing onto the slaw, stirring to coat. Taste, adjusting seasonings if necessary.
3. Cover and refrigerate to allow flavors to blend, about 2 hours.
4. Sprinkle with sesame seeds and serve.

Cranberry-Carrot Salad

Preparation Time: 15 Minutes

Cooking Time: 0 Minutes

Servings: 4

Ingredients

- 1 pound carrots, shredded
- 1 cup sweetened dried cranberries
- 2 tablespoons fresh lemon juice
- 1/2 cup toasted walnut pieces
- 3 tablespoons toasted walnut oil
- 1/8 teaspoon freshly ground black pepper

Directions

1. In a large bowl, combine the carrots, cranberries, and walnuts. Set aside.
2. In a small bowl, whisk together the lemon juice, walnut oil and pepper.
3. Pour the dressing over the salad, toss gently to combine and serve.

Mediterranean Quinoa Salad

Preparation Time: 5 Minutes

Cooking Time: 20 Minutes

Servings: 4

Ingredients

- 2 cups water
- 1 cup quinoa, well rinsed
- 2 green onions, minced
- 11/2 cups cooked or 1 (15.5-ounce) can chickpeas, drained and rinsed
- 1 cup ripe grape or cherry tomatoes, halved
- 1/2 medium English cucumber, peeled and chopped
- Salt
- 1/4 cup pitted brine-cured black olives
- 2 tablespoons toasted pine nuts
- 1/4 cup small fresh basil leaves
- 1 medium shallot, chopped
- 1 garlic clove, chopped
- 1 teaspoon Dijon mustard
- 2 tablespoons white wine vinegar

- 1/4 cup olive oil
- Freshly ground black pepper

Directions

1. In a large saucepan, bring the water to boil over high heat. Add the quinoa, salt the water, and return to a boil. Reduce heat to low, cover, and simmer until water is absorbed, about 20 minutes.
2. Transfer the cooked quinoa to a large bowl. Add the chickpeas, tomatoes, green onions, cucumber, olives, pine nuts, and basil. Set aside.
3. In a blender or food processor, combine the shallot, garlic, mustard, vinegar, oil, and salt and pepper to taste.
4. Process until well blended. Pour the dressing over the salad, toss gently to combine, and serve.

Marinated Mushroom Wraps

Preparation time: 15 minutes

cooking time: 0 minutes

servings: 2 wraps

Ingredients

- 3 tablespoons soy sauce
- 3 tablespoons fresh lemon juice
- 11/2 tablespoons toasted sesame oil
- 1 ripe tomato, chopped
- 1 ripe Hass avocado, pitted and peeled
- 2 portobello mushroom caps, cut into 1/4-inch strips
- 2 (10-inchwhole-grain flour tortillas
- 2 cups fresh baby spinach leaves
- 1 medium red bell pepper, cut into 1/4-inch strips
- Salt and freshly ground black pepper

Directions

1. In a medium bowl, combine the soy sauce, 2 tablespoons of lemon juice, and the oil. Add the portobello strips, toss to combine, and marinate for 1 hour or overnight. Drain the mushrooms and set aside.
2. Mash the avocado with the remaining 1 tablespoon of lemon juice.
3. To assemble wraps, place 1 tortilla on a work surface and spread with some of the mashed avocados. Top with a layer of baby spinach leaves.
4. In the lower third of each tortilla, arrange strips of the soaked mushrooms and some of the bell pepper strips. Sprinkle with the tomato and salt and black pepper to taste. Roll up tightly and cut in half diagonally.
5. Repeat with the remaining ingredients and serve.

Macadamia-Cashew Patties

Preparation time: 10 minutes

cooking time: 10 minutes

servings: 4 patties

Ingredients

- ¾ cup chopped macadamia nuts
- ¾ cup chopped cashews
- 1 jalapeño or other green chile, seeded and minced
- 1 medium carrot, grated
- 1 small onion, chopped
- 1 garlic clove, minced
- ¾ cup old-fashioned oats
- ¾ cup dry unseasoned bread crumbs
- 2 tablespoons minced fresh cilantro
- 1/2 teaspoon ground coriander
- 2 teaspoons fresh lime juice
- Canola or grapeseed oil, for frying
- Salt and freshly ground black pepper
- 4 sandwich rolls

- Lettuce leaves and condiment of choice

Directions

1. In a food processor, combine the macadamia nuts, cashews, carrot, onion, garlic, chile, oats, bread crumbs, cilantro, coriander, and salt and pepper to taste. Process until well mixed.
2. Add the lime juice and process until well blended.
3. Taste, adjusting seasonings if necessary. Shape the mixture into 4 equal patties.
4. In a large skillet, heat a thin layer of oil over medium heat. Add the patties and cook until golden brown on both sides, turning once, about 10 minutes total.
5. Serve on sandwich rolls with lettuce and condiments of choice.

Peppermint-Cilantro Artichoke Hearts

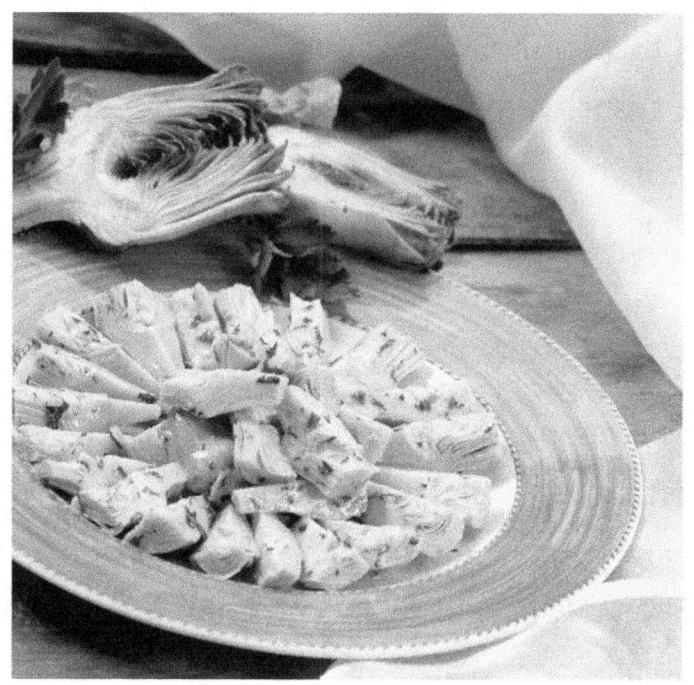

Preparation Time: 10 minutes

Cooking Time: 20 minutes

Servings: 4

Ingredients:

- 6 artichoke hearts
- 4 minced garlic cloves

- 4 tbsps. Extra-virgin olive oil
- 3 tbsps. Chopped peppermint leaves
- 3 c. water
- 3 tbsps. Chopped cilantro leaves
- 2 tbsps. Lemon juice
- Salt
- Black pepper

Directions:

1. In a deep pan place cleaned artichokes along with water, oil, cilantro leaves, peppermint, lemon juice, and garlic.
2. Season salt and pepper to taste and bring to a boil.
3. Reduce heat and simmer artichokes about 15–20 minutes, turning occasionally.
4. Transfer artichokes to a serving platter and drizzle with some of the cooking liquid.
5. Serve.

Nutrition:

Calories: 33, Fat: 13.77g, Carbs: 9.47g, Protein: 5.48

Carrot Cake Bites

Preparation Time: 15 minutes

Cooking Time: 0 minute

Servings: 15

Ingredients:

- 2 cups oats, old-fashioned
- ½ cup grated carrot
- 2 cups coconut flakes, unsweetened
- 1/2 teaspoon salt
- 1/2 teaspoon vanilla extract, unsweetened
- 1 teaspoon cinnamon
- 1/2 cup maple syrup
- 1/2 cup almond butter
- 2 tablespoons white chocolate chips

Directions:

1. Place oats in a food processor, add coconut and pulse until ground.
2. Then add remaining ingredients except for chocolate chips and pulse for 3 minutes until a sticky dough comes together.

3. Add chocolate chips, pulse for 1 minute until just mixed, and then shape the mixture into fifteen small balls.
4. Refrigerate the balls for 30 minutes and then serve.

Nutrition:

Calories: 87 Cal, Fat: 5 g, Carbs: 9.2 g, Protein: 1.8 g, Fiber: 1.6 g

Minty Fruit Salad

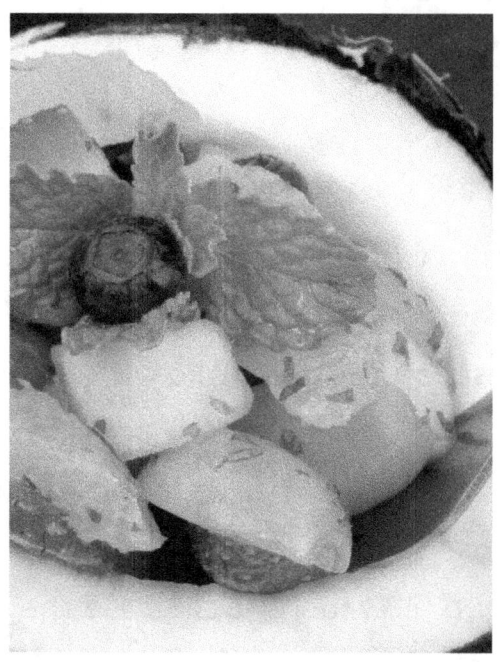

Preparation time: 15 minutes

cooking time: 5 minutes

servings: 4

Ingredients

- ¼ cup lemon juice (about 2 small lemons
- 4 teaspoons maple syrup or agave syrup
- 2 cups chopped strawberries

- 2 cups chopped pineapple
- 2 cups raspberries
- 1 cup blueberries
- 8 fresh mint leaves

Directions

1. Beginning with 1 mason jar, add the ingredients in this order:
2. 1 tablespoon of lemon juice, 1 teaspoon of maple syrup, ½ cup of pineapple, ½ cup of strawberries, ½ cup of raspberries, ¼ cup of blueberries, and 2 mint leaves.
3. Repeat to fill 3 more jars. Close the jars tightly with lids.
4. Place the airtight jars in the refrigerator for up to 3 days.

Nutrition:

Calories: 138; Fat: 1g; Protein: 2g; Carbohydrates: 34g; Fiber: 8g; Sugar: 22g; Sodium: 6mg

Avocado and Strawberries Salad

Preparation time: 5 minutes

Cooking time: 0 minutes

Servings: 4

Ingredients:

- 2 avocados, pitted, peeled and cubed
- 1 cup strawberries, halved
- 1 teaspoon almond extract
- 2 tablespoons almonds, chopped
- Juice of 1 lime
- 1 tablespoon stevia

Directions:

1. In a bowl, combine the avocados with the strawberries, and the other ingredients, toss and serve.

Nutrition:

calories 150, fat 3, fiber 3, carbs 5, protein 6

Mint Avocado Bars

Preparation time: 10 minutes

Cooking time: 25 minutes

Servings: 6

Ingredients:

- 1 teaspoon almond extract
- ½ cup coconut oil, melted
- 1 avocado, peeled, pitted and mashed
- 2 cups coconut flour
- 2 tablespoons stevia
- 1 tablespoon cocoa powder

Directions:

1. In a bowl, combine the coconut oil with the almond extract, stevia and the other ingredients and whisk well.
2. Transfer this to baking pan, spread evenly, introduce in the oven and cook at 370 degrees F and bake for 25 minutes.
3. Cool down, cut into bars and serve.

Nutrition:

calories 230, fat 12.2, fiber 4.2, carbs 15.4, protein 5.8

Coconut milk smoothie

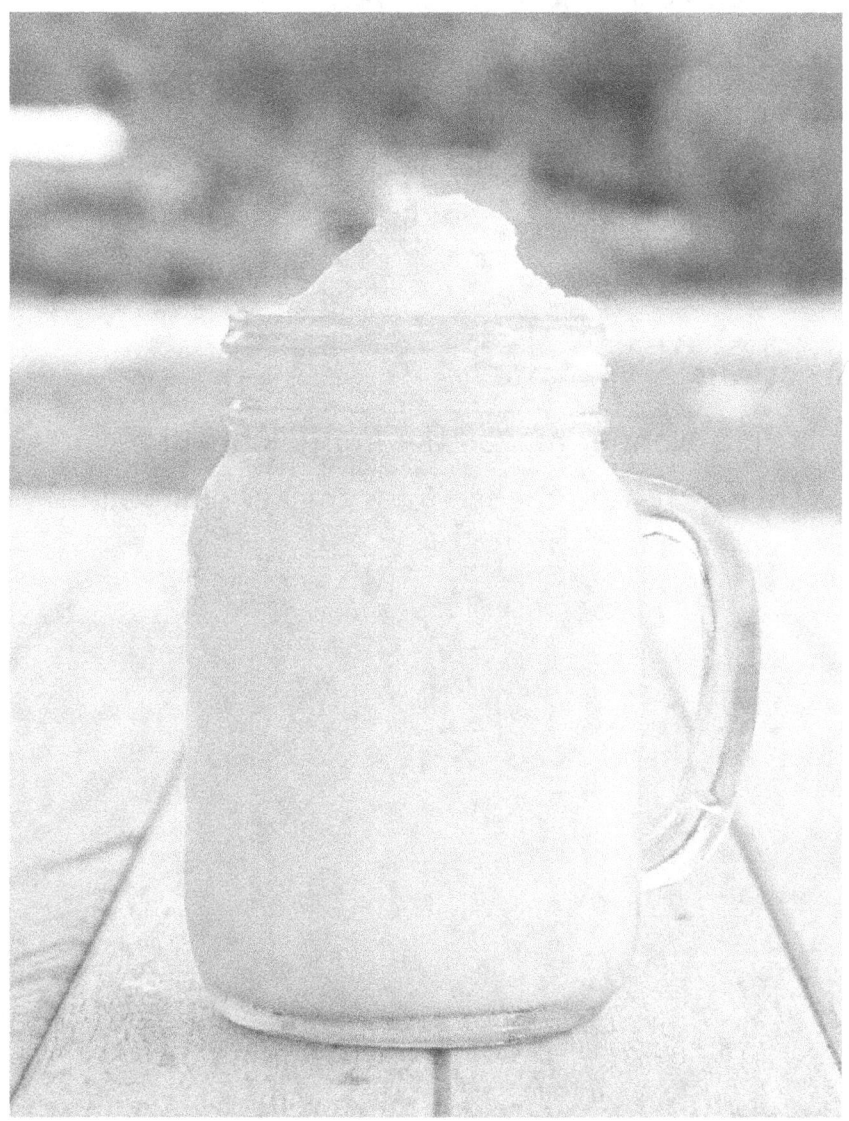

Preparation time: 15 minutes

Ingredients:

- 1 cup Greek yogurt
- 1 cup coconut milk, full fat
- 1 banana, fresh or frozen
- 1 tbsp. honey
- 1 cup baby spinach, fresh
- 5 Oz. blueberries or other berries

Directions:

1. In a blender mix all the ingredients until smooth. Add the ice for a thicker smoothie.

Keto Lemon Fat Bombs

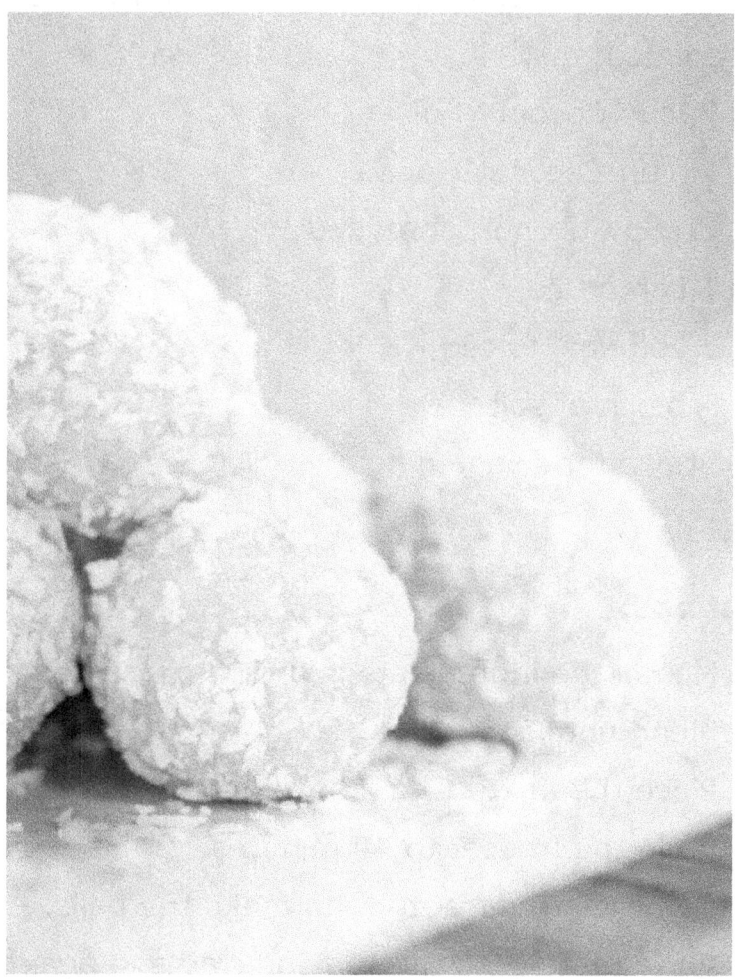

Preparation time: 60 minutes

Ingredients (for approx. 30 fat bombs):

- 1 cup Coconut Oil, melted
- 2 cups Raw Cashews, boiled for 10 minutes, soaked
- ½ cup Coconut Butter
- ¼ cup Coconut Flour
- ⅓ cup Coconut, shredded
- 1 Lemon Zest
- 2 Lemons, juiced
- A pinch of salt
- Stevia for sweetening

Directions:

1. Mix all the ingredients in a food processor and blend until combined.
2. Place the mixture to a bowl and have it cooled up in the freezer to 40 minutes.
3. Remove from freezer and make the balls.
4. Place them onto the cooking tray and again place into the freezer for hardening.
5. Remove from the freezer and store in an air-tight container for up to a week. Let them thaw before serving.

Chia Squares

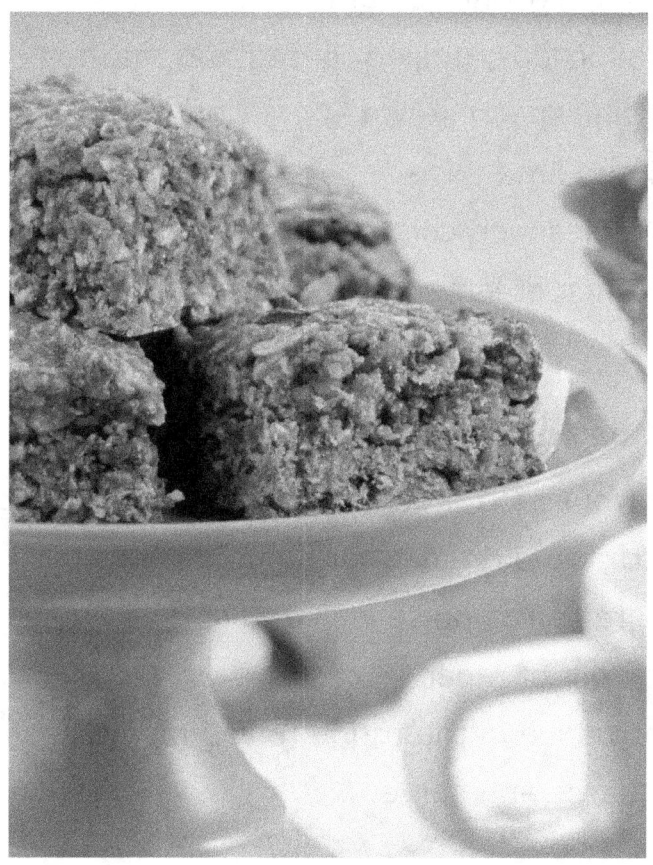

Preparation time: 30 minutes

Cooking time: 0 minutes

Servings: 4

Ingredients:

- 1 cup avocado oil
- ¼ cup coconut cream
- 2 avocados, peeled, pitted and mashed
- 1 tablespoon stevia
- ¼ cup lime juice
- 1 tablespoon chia seeds
- A pinch of lemon zest, grated

Directions:

1. In your food processor, combine the avocados with the oil, the cream and the other ingredients, pulse well and spread on the bottom of a pan.
2. Introduce in the fridge for 30 minutes, slice into squares and serve.

Nutrition:

calories 349, fat 32.5, fiber 12, carbs 15.8, protein 4.1

Mint Rice Pudding

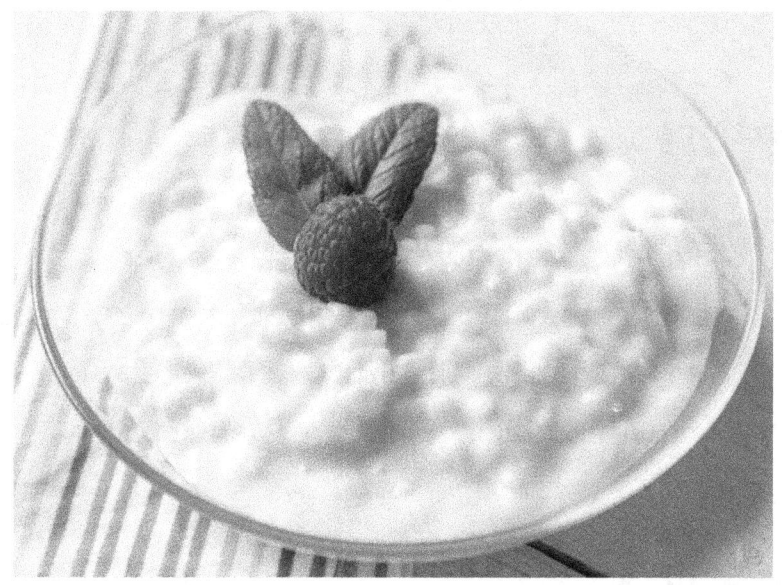

Preparation time: 10 minutes

Cooking time: 30 minutes

Servings: 4

Ingredients:

- ¼ cup stevia
- 2 cups cauliflower rice
- 2 cups coconut milk
- 2 tablespoons walnuts, chopped

- 1 tablespoon mint, chopped
- 1 teaspoon lime zest, grated
- ½ cup coconut cream

Directions:

1. In a pan, combine the cauliflower rice with the stevia, the coconut milk and the other ingredients, whisk, bring to a simmer and cook over medium-low heat for 30 minutes.
2. Divide the pudding into bowls and serve.

Nutrition:

calories 200, fat 6.3, fiber 2, carbs 6.5, protein 8

Mug Cake

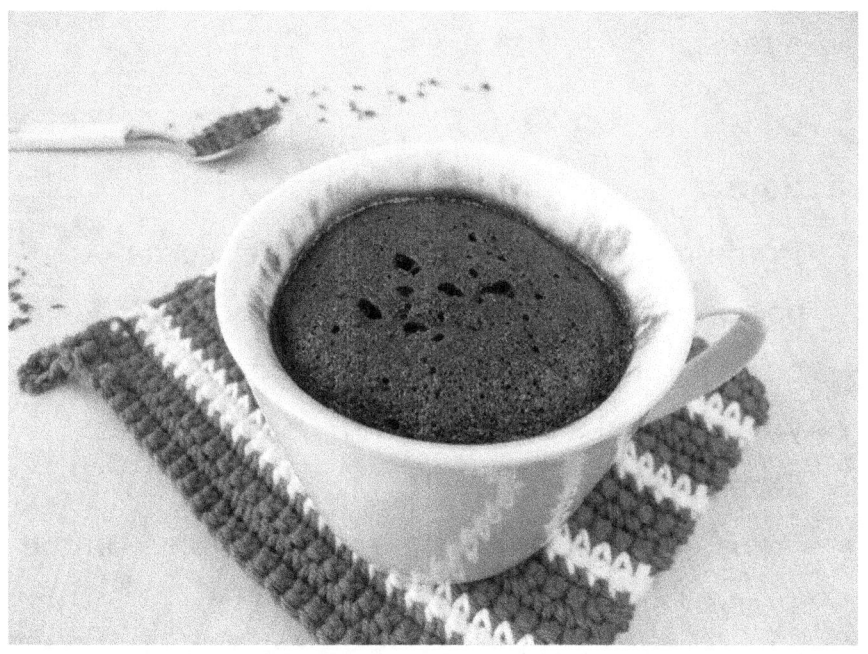

Preparation Time: 8 minutes

Cooking time: 1.5 hours

Servings: 4

Ingredients:

- 4 tablespoons pecans, chopped
- 4 teaspoon of cocoa powder
- 4 tablespoon almond flour

- ½ teaspoon baking powder
- 1 teaspoon vanilla extract
- 4 tablespoon almond milk
- 4 teaspoon Erythritol

Directions:

- In the mixing bowl mix up together cocoa powder, almond flour, vanilla extract, baking powder, almond milk, and Erythritol.
- When the mixture is smooth – add chopped pecans. Stir it.
- Transfer the batter in the mugs and place in the oven.
- Cook the mug cakes for 10 minutes on 360F.
- Eat the cakes directly from the mugs.

Nutritions:

Calories 91, fat 8.3, fiber 1.8, carbs 3.8, protein 2.1

NOTE

www.ingramcontent.com/pod-product-compliance
Lightning Source LLC
Chambersburg PA
CBHW070933080526
44589CB00013B/1495